CONTENTS

Acknowledgements

Introduction

Chapter 1   **TONSILS AND ADENOIDS**   **1**

Function
Tonsils
Adenoids

Chapter 2   **THE NOSE**   **25**

Examination
Nasal obstruction
The sinuses and sinusitis
Nose bleed
Nasal injuries

Chapter 3   **THE THROAT**   **63**

Examination
Sore throat
Dysphagia
The larynx
Tracheostomy

Chapter 4   **THE EARS**   **109**

Examination

Tests of hearing
Anatomy
Physiology
Tests of inner ear function
Diseases of the pinna
Diseases of the external
  auditory meatus
Diseases of the ear drum
Abnormalities of the middle ear
Inner ear diseases

Chapter 5   **FACIAL NERVE PARALYSIS**   **164**

Trauma
Inflammation
Tumour – acoustic neuroma
Intracranial

Chapter 6   **HEAD AND NECK CANCER**   **169**

Introduction
Individual tumours
Diagnosis of a lateral neck mass
Management of a solitary
  neck mass

ACKNOWLEDGE-MENTS

I acknowledge with gratitude all the help given to me by chiefs in the past and by my colleagues over the years who have helped to mould my ideas about ENT. They must, of course, be congratulated on the good bits of the book and not in any way blamed for the bad, for which I take full responsibility!

In particular, I would like to mention my guide and mentor, the late Mr Lionel Taylor and my wise and delightful colleague in Southampton, the late Mr Noel Morgan who died on the day on which the manuscript was sent to the publishers.

My daughter Joanna has provided me with the pens to handwrite this and other manuscripts and has encouraged me to finish my medical writing so that I can begin my novel which she assumes will make a large fortune! The typing and proof-reading were carried out with their accustomed care and skill by Mrs Glenda Young and Mrs Ann Maclellan.

J. A. S Carruth
1986

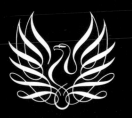

INTRODUCTION

The title of this book could/should read 'The Absolute Essentials or the Bare Necessities of ENT', 'Edited Highlights of ENT' or 'ENT for the Disinterested'.

All doctors, whether they like it or not, need to know a considerable amount about ENT. In general practice it is generally accepted that ENT problems make up more than one-third of the organic disease which is seen, and many of these problems are relatively simple disorders which nevertheless need to be treated well to avoid complications. In hospital practice many junior doctors will have under their care, by accident or design, post-tonsillectomy patients and those with tracheostomies, both demanding informed and careful management.

This book aims to cover the essentials of ENT which need to be known, and it is to be hoped that there is plenty of wood not concealed by too many trees. Serious, life-threatening conditions requiring urgent treatment are clearly identified, but little mention is made of rarities and only an outline is given of specialist management of patients once they have moved beyond first-line investigation/treatment.

The book is not comprehensive and, as such, will

offend some specialist otolaryngologists. It is based on lectures given to students, nurses, general practitioners and to the Southampton ENT FRCS course. It should appeal to all these groups and should be of value to those just beginning a career in ENT by providing 'the basics' on which specialist knowledge can be built.

CHAPTER 1

TONSILS AND ADENOIDS

Problems related to the tonsils and adenoids, and their surgical removal, make up a large and important part of ENT, both in general and hospital practice, and a majority of junior doctors will have under their care at some time, either by accident or design, post-operative T's and A's patients. It seems, therefore, appropriate to devote a chapter to them.

Function

It has been said that the only function of the tonsils is to provide Rolls Royce cars for ENT surgeons! However, many believe that they play an important role in the development of immunity.

The tonsils and adenoids form a part of Waldeyer's ring (Figure 1.1) of lymphoid tissue which surrounds the entrance to the food and air passages. The function of this lymphoid tissue is to act as a 'bacterial sampler'. A representative proportion of ingested and inspired bacteria find their way into the crypts in the lymphoid

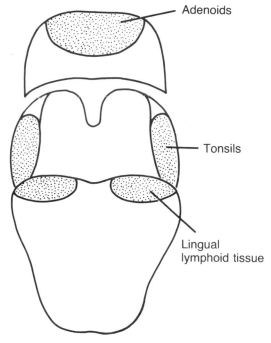

Figure 1.1   Waldeyer's ring

tissue where they are 'identified', enabling the body to produce antibodies appropriate to the bacterial environment.

Frequent attacks of tonsillitis are, therefore, inevitable when an individual enters an environment to which he has no immunity – for example, when a child first goes to school, changes class or school and when an adult changes job, boy/girl friend or moves to a new home. If a period of frequent tonsillitis is preceded by such an event it is wise to defer a decision on tonsillectomy for 12–18 months to see if the attacks naturally become less frequent.

Tonsils

Indications for tonsillectomy

In the past, tonsils were removed for minimal indications and even for social reasons and, not unreasonably, the operation got a bad name. Now, the tonsils are considered to be innocent until proved guilty, and they should only be removed for clear-cut, valid indications. When removed for these indications there can be little doubt that patients benefit significantly from the surgery and, today, the risks are infinitesimal.

Recurrent acute tonsillitis

If a patient has had more than four attacks of genuine acute tonsillitis per year, for several years, he will benefit from tonsillectomy. It is, of course, important to be certain that the attacks described by the patient are true tonsillitis and not just the sore throats which accompany a viral, upper respiratory tract infection. Each attack should last from 5 to 7 days and be accompanied by fever, enlargement of neck glands and malaise severe enough to keep the child off school or the adult away from work.

A quinsy

If a patient has had one quinsy (Figure 1.2) he is very likely to get another one unless the tonsils are removed. A quinsy is a peritonsillar abscess lying lateral to the tonsil between it and the superior constrictor muscle of the throat. It is almost always unilateral.

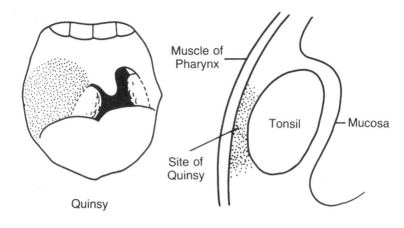

Figure 1.2   A quinsy

Symptoms

    1 Increasing pain on the affected side.

    2 Difficulty in opening the mouth (trismus).

    3 Dysphagia with drooling of saliva.

Signs

    1 Excess salivation.

    2 Foetid breath.

    3 Affected tonsil pushed towards mid-line by abscess.

Treatment

    1 In the early stages of cellulitis before pus has formed, antibiotics may be effective.

    2 If pus is present the abscess must be drained. Local anaesthetic is applied to the most promi-

nent part of the abscess – this may be of little value but at least it persuades the patient to allow the surgeon to open the abscess with either a guarded scalpel or quinsy forceps. Drainage of the abscess is unpleasant but results in immediate symptomatic relief, and antibiotics should be given for 5–7 days.

For histology

If one tonsil is abnormal – larger or harder than the other – or if it is ulcerated, it must be removed for histology. The tonsils may be involved by a lymphoma, or the mucosa covering the tonsil may be the site for a squamous carcinoma.

In a patient who has had rheumatic fever or acute glomerulonephritis

Patients who have had one of these diseases will often be treated with long-term penicillin to avoid further β-haemolytic streptococcal infection. However, some patients may develop an allergy to penicillin or may continue to get swab-proven β-haemolytic streptococcal tonsillitis. In these cases tonsillectomy may be performed at the request of the patient's paediatrician or physician.

Size

Size alone is not a common indication for tonsillectomy – well-endowed ladies do not necessarily have a mastectomy! However, on occasions, the tonsils and adenoids may be large enough to cause significant respiratory obstruction with evidence of right-sided heart strain and even failure. A very significant symptom in these cases is sleep apnoea, when a child breathes heavily and then stops breathing for many seconds. In these cases the tonsils and adenoids must be removed as a matter of urgency.

For recurrent acute tonsillitis, and after a quinsy, the patient should be told that he would benefit from tonsillectomy but not that it must be performed. The latter advice should be given for the other indications only.

Contraindications to tonsillectomy

The following contraindications are not, of course, absolute and will obviously be more relevant when the patient has one of the less vital indications for surgery.

Age

There is no upper age limit, particularly when the tonsils have to be removed for histology. In practice, one rarely removes tonsils for the other indications above the age of 30–40 years.

It is better to wait until a child is more than 4 years old before performing tonsillectomy for several reasons:

1 They tend to be uncooperative, and for psychological reasons it is better not to admit young children to hospital unless it is essential.

2 They are probably too young to have had an adequate history of recurrent acute tonsillitis to merit an operation, and the tonsils are still of value in the development of immunity.

3 All patients lose some blood during the operation and very small children do not have much blood to lose (80 cc/kg). An individual can only lose approximately 10 per cent of his blood volume acutely without developing circulatory problems, and so a 12.5 kg child can only lose 100 cc of its total volume of 1 litre without trouble.

Any other serious illness

Particularly bleeding disorders, although most can be reversed for surgery if it is essential.

A recent acute infection

In patients who refuse blood transfusions

Each surgeon must decide for himself whether he will operate on patients who absolutely refuse to have a blood transfusion should it be necessary.

In patients who have not had polio immunisation

It was found that, when polio was common, those who had just had their tonsils removed were more likely to get polio, which was often of a bulbar type, than those who had not had the operation.

The operation

Under a general anaesthetic, with an endotracheal tube in place and the mouth held open with a gag, the tonsils are peeled from the wall of the throat and only the mucosa covering the tonsils has to be cut. Blunt dissection is used to divide the adhesions between the tonsil and the superior constrictor muscle, but sharp dissection may be needed if the adhesions are excessive, as after a quinsy. Bleeding is controlled by packing the tonsillar fossae to control small vessels, and ligatures are used to tie more major vessels. Diathermy can be used, but is not popular.

Classification of haemorrhage

The only really significant complication of tonsillectomy is haemorrhage, and it can be classified into three types:

Primary haemorrhage

This occurs at the time of operation and all bleeding must be controlled by the surgeon before the patient leaves the operating table.

Reactionary haemorrhage

This occurs some hours after surgery and may be caused by a relaxation of spasm in the blood vessels within the tonsillar fossae. A factor in the control of bleeding from an acutely divided vessel is spasm with clot formation in the closed vessel end. If, when the spasm relaxes, the clot has not formed adequately or has not become adherent, then bleeding may occur. In addition, reactionary haemorrhage may occur with an increase in blood pressure in the recovery period.

Secondary haemorrhage

This occurs 5–10 days after surgery and is caused by infection in the tonsillar fossa. It will be preceded by a number of warning signs including a rise in temperature, an increase in pain – often referred to the ear – and an increase and change in the colour of the slough present in the tonsillar fossa, which is normally clean and white/yellow but will become dark and possibly haemorrhagic.

Signs of haemorrhage

It is essential that all those who are entrusted with the care of post-tonsillectomy patients are familiar with the signs of haemorrhage.

Rising pulse

All post-operative patients will be on a regular pulse chart and all will have a raised pulse which will gradually return to normal over a period of hours. However, if the pulse is rising it must be assumed that the patient is bleeding.

Appearance of the patient

A bleeding patient will be pale, cold and sweaty, an appearance described as clammy.

Blood

Blood may be visible coming from the nose or mouth, or the patient may be swallowing excessively and it must be assumed that he is swallowing blood.

Restlessness

Patients who are bleeding are apprehensive and agitated. Therefore, in the post-operative period, excessive sedation must be avoided or it will mask this important sign of restlessness.

A falling blood pressure is not a valuable measurement, particularly in children. First, the child must be woken up and may be frightened by the procedure. It is often difficult to measure the blood pressure accurately in children. Second, it is of little diagnostic value, as a child can maintain its blood pressure by increasing cardiac output and peripheral resistance to compensate for blood loss until sudden and dangerous decompensation occurs with a rapid, late fall in blood pressure.

If any signs of bleeding are found in any patient a doctor must be summoned immediately to determine first, is the child bleeding; second, from which site; and third, the severity of the bleed.

Management of post-tonsillectomy haemorrhage

Blood

Many surgeons estimate the haemoglobin and obtain the blood group of a patient before tonsillectomy and, of course, defer the operation if the patient is anaemic. If a patient is found to be bleeding, decisions about transfusion must be made immediately based on the severity of the bleed. Should blood be cross-matched? Should the patient be transfused clear fluids, uncross-matched blood or cross-matched blood? These decisions are of the utmost importance, especially in children who have a small blood volume.

Assess severity of bleed

If severe, a patient may have to be returned to the operating theatre immediately. If less severe, conservative management may be carried out.

Conservative management

1 Remove blood clot from the bleeding tonsillar fossa with blunt Luc's forceps. The clot splints open the fossa and its removal allows the muscles to contract to "nip off" blood vessels entering the fossa through the muscle wall.

2 Sit the patient up in bed to reduce the blood pressure in the head.

3 Careful sedation of the patient.

Return to the operating theatre

If conservative treatment fails the patient must have the bleeding point ligated under anaesthetic. This is an extremely dangerous procedure and must only be undertaken by experienced staff. The main danger is that the patient will vomit swallowed blood and inhale it during the induction of the anaesthetic. To overcome this danger the patient must be anaesthetised skilfully on the operating table in the head-down position.

Before the anaesthetic begins the surgeon and nurse must be scrubbed and the instruments opened with the sucker working. If the patient does vomit, disaster may still be avoided. With the patient anaesthetised, with an endotracheal tube *in situ*, the bleeding can be controlled by ligature.

Other dangers to be considered are that the patient has had a premedication, anaesthetic and post-operative sedation, and will not have cleared all these drugs. In addition, the patient has been in shock and the physiological changes which occur in shock are not immediately reversed by transfusion.

Treatment of secondary haemorrhage

First, this should be prevented by observing the warning signs: rise in temperature, increased pain and change in character in the slough in the tonsillar fossa.

When any of these signs is observed, antibiotic treatment should be given. However, many patients are discharged from hospital shortly after surgery and may not be under medical care at this time. If bleeding occurs, treatment must be with blood transfusion and antibiotics. Removal of clot is dangerous and ligation of vessels difficult as tissues in the tonsillar fossa will be necrotic and friable and will not retain the ligature.

Adenoids

In children, problems caused by the adenoids are both significant and severe, particularly the middle ear disorders from eustachian tube dysfunction. In ENT practice, adenoidectomy is certainly one of the most common operations, and without doubt one of the most important in terms of benefit to the patient.

The adenoids hypertrophy from the age of about 3–4 until they reach their largest size compared to the size of the nasopharynx, at the age of about 5–7. They then slowly decrease in size and, with growth of the nasopharynx, they become essentially insignificant by the age of 11–12 in a majority of children. Therefore conditions caused by adenoid hypertrophy will tend to be at their worst at the age of 5–7 and should then reduce gradually until about the time of puberty.

If at surgery the tonsils are to be removed, adenoidectomy will also be performed as this adds very little to the operation. However, there are indications for adenoidectomy alone, and in these cases the tonsils will not be removed unless there is also a valid indication for this procedure.

Indications for adenoidectomy

Nasal obstruction

The classic 'adenoid child' has nasal obstruction with

mouth-breathing and snoring, with, on occasions, episodes of sleep apnoea. If the symptoms are sufficiently severe, adenoidectomy will be advised, but advice must be given in the knowledge that the symptoms should resolve by about the age of puberty. The size of the adenoids may be assessed by soft tissue lateral X-ray of the nasopharynx.

Ear disease

The ear diseases caused by hypertrophy of the adenoids are by far the most important indications for surgery to the lymphatic system in children. It has been suggested from some centres that the adenoids are not particularly relevant in the aetiology of these disorders, and other centres consider that both the tonsils and adenoids should be removed in these cases. However, a majority of ENT opinion in this country considers that the adenoids are the prime aetiological factor in the development of these forms of ear disease in children.

The adenoids lie adjacent to the openings of the eustachian tubes which lead from the nasopharynx to the middle ears, and although the adenoids may not physically obstruct the eustachian tube, they can change air flow patterns which cause eustachian tube dysfunction. The adenoids can affect the eustachian tube and therefore the middle ear, in three ways:

    1 Infection.

    2 Obstruction.

    3 Obstruction plus infection.

Infection → acute otitis media

Infection ascends the eustachian tube from the adenoids during the course of an upper respiratory tract infection, and this causes the development of an abscess in the middle ear – acute otitis media.

Symptoms

1 Severe ear ache with deafness.

2 Malaise and pyrexia.

3 If untreated the ear drum may burst with discharge of pus and relief of pain. The discharge normally dries up after a few days and then the ear drum heals rapidly, but the hearing may not return to normal for 3–4 weeks.

Signs

The following changes may be seen in the ear drum in acute otitis media: (Figure 1.3).

1 Leash of blood vessels – down the handle of the malleus.→

2 Generalised redness of the ear drum.→

3 Bulging of the ear drum, most commonly in the posterior half.→

4 Perforation and discharge.

If the symptoms and signs of acute otitis media are present, the patient must be treated to prevent perforation with its complications.

Treatment

1 Antibiotics for at least 5 days – better 7 days, ideally 10 days. There is recent evidence to suggest that much shorter courses of antibiotics

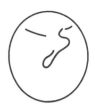

normal ear-drum

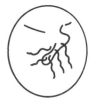

leash of blood
vessels down
malleus handle

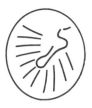

generalised
redness

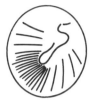

posterior half
bulges

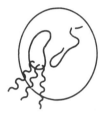

perforation

Figure 1.3   Infection → acute otitis media

may be adequate, but it is better to over-treat
rather than to treat inadequately with the risk
of rapid recurrence of the infection.

2 Nasal decongestants – to allow the infected
material to descend the eustachian tube – an
antihistamine plus nasal decongestant drops.

3 Analgesics.

4 Some favour analgesic ear drops but they are
not very widely used.

5 In the past, myringotomy – making a hole in
the ear drum – was often performed to relieve
an unresolved acute otitis media, but this is
rarely necessary today.

If a child suffers from repeated attacks of acute otitis media – three to four attacks per year for several years, particularly if the infections are accompanied by discharge – then adenoidectomy must be advised.

Obstruction → serous otitis media

The eustachian tube opens on swallowing and allows the pressure in the middle ear to equalise with atmospheric pressure.

Children with a cleft palate will suffer from eustachian tube dysfunction because the tensor palati muscle, which opens the eustachian tube, does not work normally both before and after surgery to repair the cleft.

If the eustachian tube does not open adequately, or is blocked by adenoid hypertrophy, then pressure equalisation cannot take place and the middle ear is sealed from the outside world with the following results:

1 Air is absorbed from the sealed middle ear cavity.→

2 A negative pressure develops in the middle ear.→

3 The ear drum is sucked in and cannot vibrate normally, causing slight deafness.→

4 A serous exudate is 'sucked' from the lining of the middle ear, filling the middle ear cavity and causing more severe deafness (Figure 1.4).

The deafness is severe enough to interfere with speech development and education, but as there is no ear ache or ear discharge to draw the attention of the parents to the deafness, which is often missed even by intelligent parents, the child is labelled backwards or difficult – a problem child.

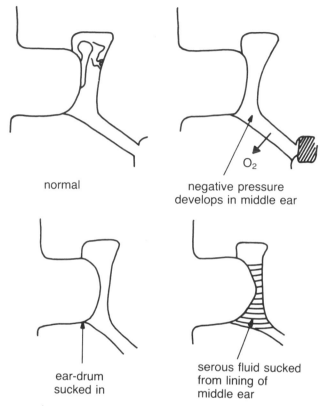

normal

negative pressure develops in middle ear

O_2

ear-drum sucked in

serous fluid sucked from lining of middle ear

Figure 1.4   Obstruction → serous otitis media

Obstruction plus infection → **glue ear** (Figure 1.5)

If, in addition to obstruction of the eustachian tube, there are also occasional episodes of infection of the middle ear, then the middle ear lining undergoes metaplasia and becomes thickened with the develop-

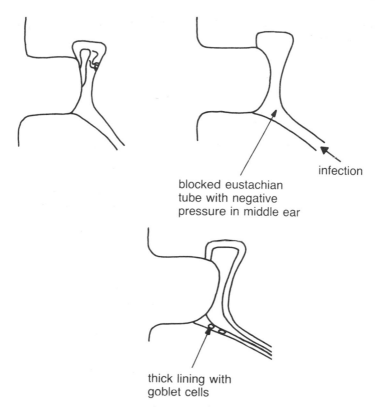

Figure 1.5   Obstruction plus infection → glue ear

ment of goblet cells which pour out a thick mucus into the middle ear. This fluid is often very thick and tenacious – hence the name "glue ear".

Symptoms of fluid in the middle ear

Deafness, may lead the child to become withdrawn, as

he cannot understand the deafness or the irritation it provokes. There may be some episodes of relatively mild ear ache in children with glue ear.

Signs of fluid in the middle ear

1 Conductive deafness.

2 The ear drum is sucked in and concave, and the handle of the malleus looks more horizontal.

3 A change in the appearance of the ear drum. The ear drum normally looks like translucent glass and light passes through it from an otoscope and is then reflected from the white medial wall of the middle ear, giving a high level of illumination in the ear canal. When examining an ear which has fluid in the middle ear, the first thought may be that the battery of the otoscope has run down, as light is absorbed by the fluid in the middle ear, and the level of illumination in the external auditory meatus is much reduced.

4 The colour of the ear drum will vary from a golden yellow in serous otitis media, in which bubbles may be seen behind the ear drum, to a dull opaque grey/white in glue ear. Whatever the abnormal colour of the ear drum, if the child does not have pain then there must be an accumulation of sterile fluid in the middle ear.

5 Occasionally there may be a leash of vessels on the handle of the malleus, which may be more obvious when the ear is manipulated or examined roughly. However, if blood vessels running radially on the surface of the ear drum are seen, this is diagnostic of fluid in the middle ear

and, as mentioned earlier, if there is no pain then this effusion is sterile.

Treatment of a child with fluid in the middle ear

Decongestant therapy

The child may be given antihistamines and nasal decongestant drops for 4–6 weeks to see if the fluid can be dispersed by improving eustachian tube function. However, many ENT surgeons are not convinced of the value of this regime and it would also be appropriate simply to watch the child over this period of time to determine the natural history of his ear disease.

Surgery

If conservative treatment fails to disperse the fluid, or if the fluid recurs regularly, then surgery must be advised or the child will suffer significantly from the persistent deafness. Adenoidectomy and myringotomy will be performed in almost all units, although some will not remove the adenoids unless they are extremely large and others will remove both the tonsils and the adenoids. At myringotomy, the fluid will be either thin in serous otitis media or thick in glue ear.

Serous Otitis Media

If the fluid is thin then the lining of the eustachian tube and middle ear will also be thin, and adenoidectomy should restore eustachian tube function.

Glue Ear

However, if the fluid is thick then the lining of the

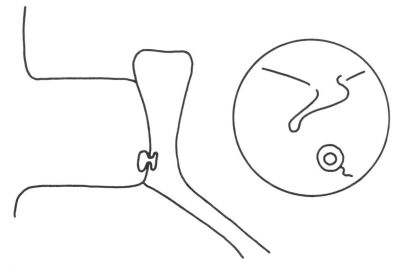

Figure 1.6   A grommet

middle ear and eustachian tube will also be thick and adenoidectomy will be unsuccessful in restoring eustachian tube function as the tube will be blocked by the thick lining and glue. In these cases a grommet will be necessary (Figure 1.6). A grommet is a small plastic bobbin with a hole through it, which acts as an artificial eustachian tube. It is inserted through a myringotomy incision like a collar stud through a button hole and is almost always inserted in the antero-inferior quadrant of the ear drum which is furthest away from vital middle ear structures and nearest to the eustachian tube. This area of the drum is the most stiff and retains the grommet better. The grommet ventilates the middle ear and will be extruded naturally after a period of some months. It is hoped that by this time the middle ear mucosa will have returned to normal with the restoration of eustachian tube function. Unfortunately this is not always the case and grommets may have to be reinserted several times.

While the grommet is *in situ* it acts as a small perforation of the ear drum and many advise children not to swim. However, recent evidence suggests that most children can swim without significant risk of infection and, if infection does occur, it shows itself by mucoid discharge from the ear which can be dried up by antibiotics and local antibiotic/steroid ear drops.

The operation

The adenoids are scraped from the base of the skull with a curette and care is taken not to damage the eustachian tube openings. The curette is fitted with a guard with teeth which catch the fragments of adenoid tissue to ensure their removal from the nasopharynx. Haemostasis is achieved by packing, and continued bleeding usually means that there are tags of adenoid tissue left behind and the nasopharynx will then be recuretted and repacked until all bleeding has ceased.

Complications of adenoidectomy

Inhalation of adenoid fragments

This can be avoided by using a guarded curette and by careful palpation and suction of the nasopharynx.

Bleeding

The signs of bleeding are the same as those described

after tonsillectomy, and the blood may be seen coming from the nose or may be swallowed. On examination, blood can be seen running down the posterior wall of the nasopharynx behind the soft palate.

Treatment of haemorrhage

As with a tonsillar haemorrhage blood transfusion is given as appropriate, and for conservative management the patient is sat up and sedated. If the bleeding does not stop a post-nasal pack must be inserted.

The classical technique for inserting a gauze pack, which must be carried out under a general anaesthetic in children, is described in the section on nose bleeding. However, it is much easier and kinder to use a fine bladder catheter with a 30 cc balloon. This is passed along the floor of the nose after lubrication and surface anaesthetic of the nasal mucosa. When the balloon is in the nasopharynx it can be inflated, and the pressure will control the bleeding. This procedure can be carried out without a general anaesthetic even in nervous children.

CHAPTER 2

THE NOSE

Examination

First, the external appearance of the nose must be assessed and then the inside of the nose can be examined using the electric auroscope with a large speculum but without the magnifying lens, which would become misted.

After examining the nasal vestibule for infection, the nasal mucosa should be assessed. This is normally a pink/red colour but may be a blue/violet colour in nasal allergy and will be much more hyperaemic in cases of nasal and sinus infection. The nasal septum should be essentially central but is rarely totally straight and usually has some slight cartilaginous or bony irregularities. The turbinates are fleshy cylinders attached to the lateral walls of the nose and the whole of the inferior turbinate can usually be seen, but only the inferior half of the middle turbinate is visible.

It is often possible to mistake a swollen turbinate for a polyp, but a polyp is usually paler in colour than the nasal mucosa and, if palpated with an orange stick or probe, it will move and will not be sensitive, whereas a turbinate is obviously immobile and is extremely sensitive to the touch.

Nasal Obstruction

Structural abnormalities

Deviated nasal septum

Aetiology

Congenital or traumatic.

Symptoms

Blockage of nose on side of convexity.

Signs

Deviation of cartilaginous and/or bony nasal septum.

Treatment

Submucous resection of the nasal septum (SMR, Figure 2.1). The cartilage and bone of the nasal septum are covered on either side by perichondrium and periosteum and nasal mucosa. In the operation the mucoperiosteum/perichondrium is elevated from the bone and cartilage on both sides of the septum, and deviated bone and cartilage is removed. A strip of cartilage must be left in the nasal bridge to prevent collapse and in the columella at the root of the nose, to

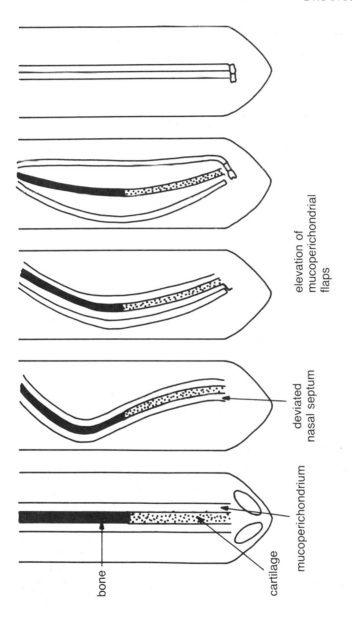

elevation of
mucoperichondrial
flaps

deviated
nasal septum

mucoperichondrium

bone

cartilage

Figure 2.1   The SMR operation

prevent retraction with 'beaking'. Care must be taken not to perforate the mucoperichondrial flaps on both sides or a permanent perforation will result. If this is small, the perforation whistles, and if large, crusting and bleeding occurs. Septal perforations are extremely difficult to repair.

Choanal atresia

Aetiology

Congenital failure of the posterior nasal aperture (posterior choana) to cannalise.

Symptoms

In cases of bilateral complete choanal atresia, severe problems may develop in the child at birth as the neonate will not breathe through its mouth. Periods of cyanosis may occur – cyclical cyanosis of the newborn – and death has been reported.

Urgent treatment to perforate the obstructing partition must be carried out, and an indwelling plastic nasal airway must be left *in situ*. Once the emergency is over, the obstructing partition may be removed, either transnasally using the carbon dioxide surgical laser, or surgically through the palate.

Unilateral choanal atresia presents with complete obstruction on the affected side and clear, glassy mucoid discharge. Transpalatal surgery will be carried out in these cases.

Foreign body

Children insert a wide range of objects into the nose.

Although nasal obstruction will be present the main symptom and sign is a foul, unilateral or bilateral nasal discharge.

It may be possible to remove the foreign bodies in the general practitioner's surgery, but many will need referral to an ENT clinic, where good illumination for the examination of the nose and appropriate instruments are available. The majority can be removed without a general anaesthetic from cooperative or firmly restrained children, but on occasions a general anaesthetic will be necessary.

Changes in the nasal mucosa

The response of the nasal mucosa to all insults is essentially similar. Sneezing attempts to blow away the irritant and watery nasal discharge attempts to wash it away. Oedema and hyperaemia of the nasal mucosa cause obstruction.

Inflammation

Acute viral

The common cold, influenza and the prodromal symptoms of the infectious fevers cause the symptoms of blockage, discharge and sneezing. Treatment is symptomatic.

Bacterial

An acute boil may occur in the nasal vestibule in the hair-bearing area. Antibiotic treatment will usually be successful but drainage may be needed.

Vestibulitis is common in children due to mild nasal trauma from picking, and it may be secondary to anterior nasal discharge. A simple antibiotic cream will usually clear this infection.

Acute and chronic bacterial rhinitis is almost always part of an infection of the nose and maxillary sinuses, and its diagnosis and management are discussed in the section on sinusitis.

Nasal allergy

This is a complex and fascinating problem and the treatment suggested in this chapter represents simple, practical measures which should help many patients. Others will require more complex, specialist investigation and treatment.

The changes in the nasal mucosa are provoked by histamine released from mast cells in the mucosa when provoked by the allergen.

For the purpose of management, nasal allergy may be divided into two groups:

  1 Acute paroxysmal.

  2 Perennial.

Acute paroxysmal

Symptoms

Acute episodes of 'allergic nasal symptoms' with sneezing, blockage and watery nasal discharge when provoked by a specific allergen – pollen, fur, feathers, etc. Between paroxysmal attacks the patient is symptom-free and the nose is relatively normal, but in an acute episode the nasal mucosa is oedematous and often has a blue/purple colour. Watery, mucoid discharge is present in the nasal cavities. Specific allergens can readily be identified on skin testing.

Treatment

The acute attack

1 Antihistamines.

2 Disodium cromoglycate which stabilises the mast cells.

3 A steroid nasal spray.

Desensitisation

This is of great value for classical hay fever or for specific paroxysmal allergies. The patient is injected with gradually increasing doses of the allergen, to build up resistance. However, the course of injections is not pleasant and may be accompanied by severe systemic reactions.

Perennial allergy

In this condition the patient complains of allergic symptoms which persist throughout the year, and are less severe and dramatic than those with the acute paroxysmal allergies.

Symptoms

Perennial obstruction, watery discharge and sneezing.

Signs

Oedematous mucosa which is blue/violet in colour.

Diagnosis

The patient usually has a weak positive response to a large number of allergens on skin testing.

Treatment

Desensitisation injections are rarely of benefit for patients with perennial nasal allergy. However, within this group are patients with an allergy to the house dust mite. Avoidance of dusty conditions and specific precautions around the house will decrease this problem, and a number of patients with this allergy can obtain benefit from desensitising injections.

1 Antihistamines may be of value, but they have unpleasant side-effects.

2 Disodium cromoglycate is of great help in asthma and paroxysmal allergy but is of limited value in perennial cases, although some find it to be a great help.

3 Low-dose steroid nasal sprays. These sprays have revolutionised the management of these cases, as they appear to be without significant side-effects and there is no rebound vasodilatation after use, as there is with the decongestant sprays.

4 If conservative treatment fails the patient may need surgery. The surgery will depend on the major symptom, which will be either blockage or severe, watery nasal discharge.

    (a) Blockage – the swollen, hypertrophid turbinates may be treated by cautery or submucosal diathermy to cause shrinkage or they may be reduced in size surgically, with great care. A delicate equation exists within the nose – the nasal mucosa attempts to warm and humidify the inspired air and the inspired air dries and cools the nasal mucous membrane. If too much mucosa is removed, the equation moves in the wrong direction and the mucosa becomes dry and atrophic with the development of crusts which rapidly become infected and offensive – atrophic rhinitis.

It is easy to do nasal surgery badly; it is much more difficult to do it skilfully and well.

(b) Watery nasal discharge – it is rare for the symptoms to be sufficiently severe to justify surgery, but on occasions it is necessary to divide the parasympathetic nerve supply to the nasal mucosa. The vidian nerve is found in the pterygo-palatine fossa, behind the maxillary antrum. The antrum is opened by a standard sub-labial approach and the posterior wall of the antrum removed to expose the fossa and the vidian nerve is diathermised in its canal.

Vasomotor rhinitis (VMR)

This condition is difficult to define but could be called allergic rhinitis with no allergen. The allergic symptoms are perennial and produced by changes in weather, humidity, atmospheric pollution, etc.

The symptoms and signs are the same as for perennial nasal allergy, and the management is essentially the same.

Drugs

Excessive use of decongestant sprays may provoke dependence on them. The immediate vasoconstriction is followed by a reactive hyperaemia causing more nasal obstruction necessitating the use of more drops, with the development of a vicious circle. Nasal decongestant drops should not be used for more than a few weeks, but are of very great value in acute conditions. The low-dose steroid nasal sprays seem not to have this problem.

Nasal polypi

Aetiology

Nasal polypi appear to be a manifestation of nasal allergy. Polypi arise in the ethmoid air sinuses and then prolapse beneath the middle turbinates into the nose. They are not tumours but are merely bags of oedematous nasal mucosa containing tissue fluid with numerous eosinophils. They do not become malignant.

Symptoms

   1 Nasal obstruction, which is almost invariably bilateral.

   2 Watery nasal discharge.

   3 Polypi rarely cause bleeding.

Signs

Pale oedematous polypi in both sides of the nose. They are often mistaken for oedematous turbinates but if a polyp is probed it will move and is painless, whereas a turbinate obviously will not move and is extremely sensitive.

Treatment

It is easy to remove nasal polypi under either local or general anaesthetic using snares and a variety of nasal forceps. Polypi tend to recur, and in some patients this recurrence may be at intervals of only a few months. At present there is no reliable way of preventing this recurrence and although steroids, ACTH and surgical exenteration of the ethmoid air cells have all been tried, none has given consistently satisfactory results.

Nasal tumours

Benign

Adenoids

These are not, of course, 'tumour tissue'. However, physiological hypertrophy of the adenoids is by far the commonest cause of significant nasal obstruction in children.

Fibroangioma

A rare, benign tumour of the postnasal space which occurs commonly in adolescent males. It presents with blockage of the nose and bleeding, biopsy and surgery are dangerous as haemorrhage can be severe. Treatment is by radiotherapy and/or surgery may be necessary which will often be preceded by ligation of the external carotid artery and embolisation of major feeding vessels to the tumour.

Premalignant — transitional cell papilloma (inverted papilloma, Ringertz tumour)

These tumours present as 'nasal polypi' but may be

unilateral, and unilateral polypi must always be viewed with suspicion. The symptoms are similar – namely, nasal obstruction with watery nasal discharge – but haemorrhage is more common than with allergic nasal polypi. On examination they appear more fleshy and often have a granular surface. These tumours may arise either in the nasal cavity or in the sinuses and invade adjacent nose and sinus cavities by pressure erosion. Diagnosis is confirmed by histology, and although these tumours are at first benign, there is a slight but definite tendency for them to become malignant.

Treatment

The tumour must be excised completely from the nasal cavity and any affected sinuses. If surgery is imperfect there is a high chance of recurrence and careful follow-up is essential.

Malignant granuloma

In this rare group of conditions the upper air passages are involved by granulation tissue which is locally destructive. There are two main forms of the disease: first, Stewart's, in which the granulation tissue is locally very destructive; second, Wegener's granulomatosis, in which the granulation tissue is locally less aggressive but it is associated with a systemic polyarteritis which may affect the lungs and kidneys.

Treatment

The local manifestations may be treated by irradiation and systemic manifestations by steroids and chemotherapy.

Malignant tumours

Maxilla, nasal cavity and ethmoid sinuses

Aetiology

Almost always unknown, except in certain groups of woodworkers who have an unusually high incidence of ethmoidal tumours.

Pathology

Almost always squamous carcinoma but other rare tumours do occur, including secondary tumours and malignant melanomas, which tend to be less aggressive than these tumours of the skin.

Symptoms

These depend on which wall of the maxillary/ethmoid sinuses is broached by tumour. (Figure 2.2)

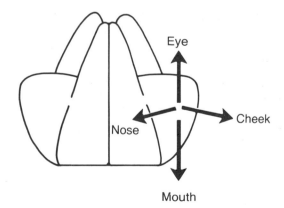

Figure 2.2   Spread of carcinoma of the maxilla

1 Nose – bleeding and blockage.

2 Mouth – toothache and, if a tooth is extracted the tumour may come through the socket. Tumour may also present through the palate or in the sulcus between the upper teeth and cheek.

3 Cheek – swelling (maxillary sinusitis does not cause swelling of the cheek).

4 Eye – proptosis, diplopia, blindness.

Signs

Evidence of tumour in the nose, cheek, mouth or orbit. It is rare for this tumour to metastasise to lymph nodes in the neck, and if they are involved it is thought by many that the tumour is then incurable.

Investigations

1 Sinus X-ray.

2 Sinus tomograms to show the extent of destruction of the bony walls of the sinuses.

3 CT scan.

4 Biopsy, either of tumour in the nasal cavity or mouth, or of tumour in the sinus via an intranasal antrostomy. It is believed by many that a Caldwell–Luc approach should not be used as this may disseminate tumour into the tissues of the cheek.

Treatment

Patients will receive a full dose of radiotherapy to 6000 rad and the orbit must be included in the field of radiation if it is involved by tumour. If the patient is fit for surgery there is evidence to show that elective surgery following radiotherapy will result in improved 'cure rates'. For tumours low in the maxilla, the hard palate on the affected side will be removed and a partial maxillectomy carried out through this palatal fenestration. For tumours higher in the maxilla and ethmoids, an external incision will be necessary and the whole maxilla removed with or without exenteration of the orbit. After both forms of surgery the defect in the hard palate will be closed by a dental plate, and on this will be mounted an obturator which fills out the defect in the cheek. When healing is complete the patient should have no trouble in talking and swallowing, there should be no asymmetry of the face and the cosmetic deformity should be limited to the carefully repaired incision on the face when this has been necessary. However, these tumours tend to present relatively late and 'cure rates' are poor.

Tumours of the postnasal space

Aetiology

Unknown, apart from some racial tendencies.

Pathology

Commonly a squamous carcinoma although a lymphoma in adenoid remnants may occur.

Symptoms

1 Sixty per cent of cases present with a metastatic lymph node high in the neck, with no symptoms from the primary tumour.

2 Serous otitis media from eustachian tube obstruction. Unilateral persistent serous otitis media in an adult must be assumed to be caused by a carcinoma of the nasopharynx until proved otherwise.

3 Nasal obstruction and bleeding.

4 Erosion of skull base with pain and cranial nerve involvement.

Signs

Neck mass, tumour in nasopharynx, serous otitis media, cranial nerve lesion.

Investigation

Base of skull X-rays to show erosion. Biopsy.

Treatment

Radiotherapy to 6000 rad. If radiotherapy fails, surgery is rarely possible, but palliation may be achieved by the use of cryotherapy or the carbon dioxide laser.

The Sinuses and Sinusitis

Acute infection of the sinuses requires skilful management to prevent the development of chronic sinusitis and urgent treatment is necessary, in acute ethmoid sinusitis with orbital cellulitis, to prevent damage to the optic nerve and, in acute frontal sinusitis, to prevent potentially fatal intracranial complications.

Acute sinusitis develops during an upper respiratory tract infection with fever, malaise and pain, with tenderness over the affected sinus or sinuses.

The pain of sinusitis is made worse by increasing venous pressure by bending or straining and often has a characteristic diurnal rhythm. The pain may be absent on waking (unlike the pain caused by raised intracranial pressure), it gets worse in the middle of the day and afternoon and tends to get better in the evening.

The pressure of pus may be considerable in an acutely infected sinus, and in the frontal and ethmoid sinuses the weakest wall may burst leading to severe extra-sinus complications. In the ethmoids the lateral wall bursts releasing pus into the orbit, and the posterior wall of the frontal sinuses bursts giving rise to intracranial complications which may develop rapidly before the patient has sought medical advice (Figure 2.3).

Lateral wall of ethmoids bursts

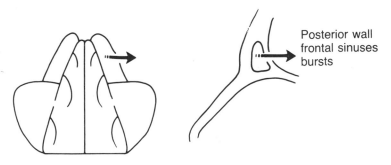

Posterior wall frontal sinuses bursts

Figure 2.3   Direction of rupture of weak sinus walls

The Sinuses (Figure 2.4)

Sphenoid

These sinuses lie in the midline at the top of the back of the nasal septum and they are of little clinical importance but occasionally an acute infection may give rise to a deep, central headache. Very rarely infection or a mucocoele of the sphenoids may involve the optic chiasma, pituitary or cavernous sinuses which lie above them. The sphenoids are most often opened by ENT surgeons during trans-sphenoidal hypophysectomy.

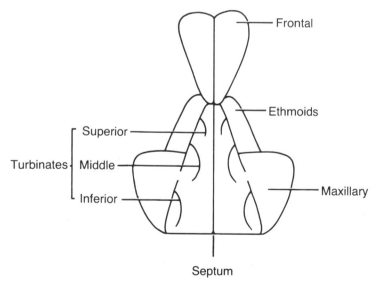

Figure 2.4   The sinuses

Frontal

Anatomy

These sinuses are contained within the frontal bones of the forehead and are not present at birth but develop in childhood. The posterior wall is the weakest.

Acute frontal sinusitis

This is a medical emergency and intracranial complications may develop with frightening rapidity. The weak posterior wall may rupture leading to meningitis, extradural abscess or brain abscess.

Symptoms

1 Severe frontal headache with the typical features of sinus pain described above.

2 Fever and malaise.

3 Nasal blockage and discharge.

Signs

1 Tenderness on percussion of the affected sinus or on pressure on the floor of the sinus at the medial end of the roof of the orbit.

2 Red nasal mucosa with pus.

Investigations

1 Nasal swab.

2 Sinus X-ray – this will show opacity of the affected sinus and almost always infection of the maxillary sinus on the same side.

Treatment

Acute frontal sinusitis is a medical emergency and treatment must be given urgently – ideally in hospital.

1 Antibiotics.

2 Nasal decongestants.

3 Sinus washout of infected maxillary antrum under local anaesthetic.

4 If the symptoms do not resolve rapidly the sinus must be drained. Under general anaesthetic through a curved incision beneath the medial end of the eye brow, the floor of the frontal sinus is opened with a gouge or drill and two fine plastic tubes are inserted into the sinus and sewn in place. The sinus is irrigated daily via one tube with warm, sterile saline which returns through the second tube. After a few days the irrigating fluid drains into the nose, indicating that the fronto-nasal duct has reopened and the tubes can be removed.

Recurrent acute frontal sinusitis and after intracranial complications

In these cases the drainage of the frontal sinus must be improved to prevent further recurrence with its attendant risks. Two operations are commonly used.

Fronto-ethmoidectomy

An incision is made beneath the medial end of the eyebrow, the periosteum of the medial wall of the orbit is elevated and the lacrymal sac displaced from the lacrymal fossa. The ethmoid air cells are entered via the lacrymal fossa and exenterated, and the middle turbinate is excised. The floor of the frontal sinus is opened widely and a large-diameter plastic tube is passed from the nose into the frontal sinuses and sewn in place for 6–8 weeks to ensure permanent drainage. (Figure 2.5)

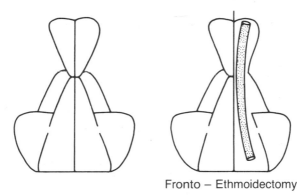

Fronto – Ethmoidectomy

Figure 2.5   The operation of fronto-ethmoidectomy

Macbeth operation

An incision from ear to ear is made over the top of the head and the forehead is turned forwards. The anterior wall of the frontal sinuses is freed by drill and turned downwards as an osteoplastic flap. The sinuses are then cleaned and the fronto-nasal ducts widened. The bone and forehead are then replaced.

Frontal sinus mucocoele

If a frontonasal duct becomes blocked – often after trauma – a mucocoele may develop and this will erode the floor of the sinus presenting as a smooth, hard swelling above the inner canthus of the eye. The patient will complain of diplopia and the diagnosis is made by X-ray. Treatment is by fronto-ethmoidectomy.

Ethmoids

Anatomy

These sinuses are made up of a chain of bony 'cells' leading from the lacrymal fossa to the sphenoid sinus lying between the nose and the orbit.

Acute ethmoid sinusitis

The lateral wall of the ethmoid sinuses is extremely thin – the lamina papyracea – and pus may burst through this into the orbit causing an extraperiosteal abscess with risk to the optic nerve.

Symptoms

1 Fever and malaise.

2 Pain and swelling around the eye.

3 Diplopia and loss of vision may occur later.

Signs

1 Orbital cellulitis with red swollen lids and chemosis.

2 Decreased eye movements and decreased visual acuity may occur later.

Investigations

1 The sinus X-ray will show opacity of the

ethmoids and almost invariably of the maxillary antrum on the same side.

2 Nasal swab.

Treatment

1 Early cases may respond to antibiotics and nasal decongestants.

2 Sinus washout of the infected maxillary antrum under local anaesthetic.

3 If the symptoms and signs do not rapidly resolve, the abscess must be drained either intranasally or externally.

It is often possible to open the ethmoid air cells adequately through the nose beneath the middle turbinate to provide satisfactory drainage. However, on occasions the abscess may have to be drained externally via an incision beneath the lower eye lid.

Nasal polypi

Pathology

These are thought to be a manifestation of nasal allergy, and they are bags of oedematous nasal mucosa containing tissue fluid with many eosinophils. They develop in the ethmoid sinuses and prolapse into the nose beneath the middle turbinate. Secondary sinusitis may develop from obstruction of sinus ostia by the polypi.

Symptoms

1 Bilateral nasal obstruction.

2 Watery nasal discharge.

3 They rarely, if ever, bleed.

4 Symptoms of sinusitis secondary to obstruction of the ostia.

Signs

1 The presence of grey, pale swellings on both sides of the nose.

2 These are not sensitive to gentle pressure with a probe, unlike the turbinates which are extremely sensitive.

3 Unilateral 'polypi' must be viewed with suspicion and may be transitional cell papillomata or other more sinister tumours.

Treatment

Under either local or general anaesthetic, the polypi are removed by snare and forceps. This is a difficult operation to perform well, and even after thorough surgery recurrence is common. The interval between surgery and recurrence varies from patient to patient and many methods have been tried to prevent recurrence but with limited success.

1 Steroids.

2 ACTH

3 Surgical exenteration of the ethmoids.

Maxillary

Anatomy

The maxillary antra lie in the cheeks, lateral to the

nose and below the orbit. The teeth in the upper alveolus lie in close proximity to the floor.

The ostium which drains the sinus is small and lies high up on the medial wall beneath the middle turbinate. The blanket of mucus from the sinus has to be carried by the cilia of the respiratory mucosa which lines the sinus in an anti-gravity direction to the ostium.

Acute maxillary sinusitis

Pathology

During an upper respiratory tract infection the ostium may become blocked and the cilia become paralysed, causing retention of mucus in the sinus which becomes infected, resulting in an abscess in the antrum. Dental infection of and/or treatment to the upper teeth, particularly the pre-molars and molars, may also lead to maxillary sinusitis.

Symptoms

1 Pain in the cheek – the patient often indicates the site of the pain by drawing a finger from the inner canthus onto the cheek. The patient may also complain of toothache.

2 Fever and malaise.

3 Nasal blockage and discharge.

Signs

1 Pain on percussion of the cheek or the teeth.

2 Red nasal mucosa with pus.

3 *No* swelling of the cheek which occurs in apical infection of the upper incisor teeth, skin infection of the cheek and rarely, carcinoma of the maxilla.

Investigation

1 Sinus X-ray will show opacity of the infected sinus with or without a fluid level.

2 Nasal swab.

Treatment

1 Antibiotics and decongestants.

2 Sinus washout is *not* performed in the acute phase as there is some danger of spreading the infection into the bone of the maxilla. However, it may be performed after some days of antibiotic treatment to remove residual non-infected mucopus from the sinus.

Recurrent acute maxillary sinusitis

A patient suffers from repeated attacks of acute maxillary sinusitis with each upper respiratory tract infection, but after treatment the nose returns to normal and remains normal between attacks.

Treatment

Each attack is treated on merit and surgery will be performed to provide permanent drainage of the sinus at its most dependent part.

Intranasal antrostomy (Figure 2.6) is performed – under a general anaesthetic with the nose cocainised, a window is created from the nose into the sinus under the inferior turbinate.

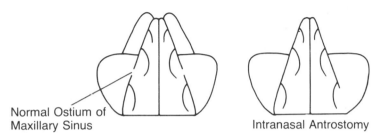

Normal Ostium of Maxillary Sinus

Intranasal Antrostomy

Figure 2.6   The operation of intranasal antrostomy

Chronic maxillary sinusitis

Pathology

Imperfectly treated acute sinusitis may result in chronic damage to the sinus lining and eventually the lining will become irreversibly damaged. Dental treatment to the pre-molars or molars may result in tooth fragments being pushed into the sinus. Chronic maxillary sinusitis may be associated with bronchiectasis.

Symptoms

1 Heaviness in the cheeks.

2 Mucopurulent postnasal drip – the infected mucus is carried backwards by the cilia of the nasal mucous membrane.

3 Nose bleeds.

4 Pharyngitis, laryngitis, bronchitis.

Signs

    1 Mucopus in the postnasal space may be visible behind the soft palate when the patient gags.

    2 Red nasal mucosa.

    3 Prominent lymphoid tissue on the posterior pharyngeal wall – granular pharyngitis.

Investigations

Sinus X-ray will show an opaque sinus with or without a fluid level. The fluid level is confirmed by X-raying the patient tipped to one side, when the fluid level will remain horizontal.

Treatment

    1 When seen in hospital further medical treatment will probably *not* be appropriate as the patient will have received a wide range of antibiotics/decongestant treatment from his general practitioner.

    2 Sinus washout will be performed. A trocar and cannula are introduced under local anaesthetic into the sinus beneath the inferior turbinate. The trocar is removed and pus is washed out of the sinus with warm, sterile saline. When the sinus has been thoroughly washed, fluid should not be displaced from the sinus by air as there is a slight risk of air embolism. The pus is cultured.

    The procedure is not pleasant but should be totally painless, if the nose has been correctly anaesthetised. Momentary distress is caused by the 'crunch' of bone as the trocar and cannula perforate the bony naso-antral wall.

The patient is given a course of appropriate antibiotics and decongestants for 2 weeks and then is reassessed.

If the symptoms have improved, further decongestants will be given. If the symptoms persist a sinus washout will be performed.

If pus is still present but much reduced from the previous washout, further antibiotic treatment will be given. However, if thick pus persists it indicates the lining of the sinus is irreversibly damaged and it must, therefore, be removed and a Caldwell–Luc procedure will be performed.

Under general anaesthetic an incision is made in the upper gum above the roots of the incisor–premolar teeth, the soft tissues of the cheek are elevated and retracted and the anterior wall of the sinus opened with hammer and gouge. The lining of the sinus is then removed and a large window made from nose to sinus beneath the inferior turbinate to provide permanent, dependent drainage.

The clean well-drained sinus will then be recolonised by healthy respiratory mucosa.

In the past, multiple sinus washouts were performed weekly for many weeks, but this is now thought to be inappropriate. However, the Caldwell–Luc operation is performed with decreasing frequency for chronic sinusitis.

Antro-choanal polyp

This uncommon polyp (Figure 2.7) develops within the maxillary sinus and the polyp is then drawn to the osteum by the cilia and then backwards into the naso-pharynx. It causes at first unilateral, and subse-

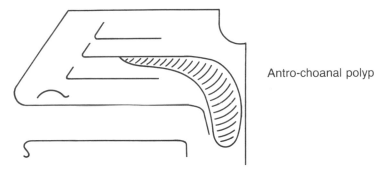

Antro-choanal polyp

Figure 2.7   Antro-choanal polyp

quently bilateral, nasal obstruction. The polyp may be visible behind the soft palate when the patient gags, or on rare occasions at rest. It is readily visible with a postnasal mirror.

A sinus X-ray will show an opaque antrum with the classical diffuse opacity – the ground-glass appearance.

Treatment is by polypectomy and the stalk is removed from the antrum by a Caldwell–Luc procedure. Polypectomy alone will be performed in the young patient when the upper teeth have not erupted, as these unerupted teeth may be damaged during the opening of the antrum. On occasions polypectomy alone will be carried out in very elderly patients.

Nose Bleed

Aetiology

Trauma, hypertension, nasal infection, sinusitis, bleeding disorders; in children, minor trauma and vestibulitis with bleeding from Little's area, where there is a confluence of vessels at the anterior part of the nasal septum.

Symptoms

A nose bleed varies in severity from a trivial inconvenience to a life-threatening disaster.

Treatment

Blood replacement

The 'circulatory status' of the patient must be constantly assessed during any significant haemorrhage, and appropriate replacement carried out.

To control the bleeding

Trotter's method (Figure 2.8)

1 Sit the patient up to reduce blood pressure in the head.

2 Lean the patient forward to avoid swallowing blood and to assess the severity of bleed.

3 Provide a bowl to catch the blood.

4 Place an object between the patient's teeth to ensure mouth-breathing.

If Trotter's method has been tried unsuccessfully for a period of time determined by the severity of the bleed and the tolerance of the patient, the soft anterior parts of the nose may be compressed for several minutes between finger and thumb, and cold compresses may

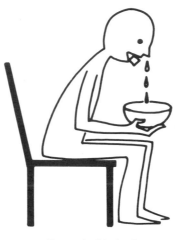

Trotter's Method

Figure 2.8   Trotter's method

be applied to the bridge of the nose and/or back of the neck.

If this fails *the nose must be examined*; this requires a good light and head mirror, soft rubber catheters with gentle suction and protective clothing for the examiner. If the nose is examined, the patient tends to sneeze, covering the examiner with a fine spray of blood!

If the bleeding point can be seen it will be cauterized under local anaesthetic with an electric cautery. Chemical cautery is possible, but active bleeding makes this difficult as the blood tends to wash away the chemical.

If the bleeding point cannot be seen the nose must be packed (Figure 2.9) and to do this successfully, careful local anaesthetic must be applied.

1 Traditionally the nose is packed with ½ inch (13

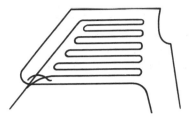

nasal packing with ribbon gauze

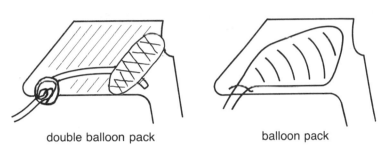

double balloon pack   balloon pack

Figure 2.9   Nasal packing

mm) or 1 inch (25 mm) *ribbon gauze* introduced with nasal packing forceps, layer upon layer from the floor of the nose until the nasal cavity is filled and the bleeding controlled. The pack must not be moistened with a water-based preparation as this will dry out in the nose and make removal of the pack difficult and traumatic. Usually ribbon gauze impregnated with BIPP (bismuth iodoform paraffin paste) is used. Bismuth is haemostatic, iodoform keeps the pack clean in the nose, and paraffin lubricates the pack. If this is not available the gauze may be impregnated with liquid paraffin or glycerine, but excess 'liquid' must be removed before the pack is introduced, to avoid inhalation.

If a pack is left *in situ* for more than 24 hours, *antibiotics must be given* or the pack will become infected.

2 *Inflatable rubber packs* may be used if available. Packing with ribbon gauze is difficult for the inexperienced, but the various forms of inflatable pack which are available are both effective and easy to insert even with minimal local anaesthetic. A simple pack may be constructed by tying a finger stall onto a catheter, but ready-made packs of various designs are available, either to fill the nasal cavity or to plug the anterior and posterior openings from the nose, allowing the blood in nose to 'pack it'.

3 *Postnasal packing* will be needed if, after an anterior pack has been inserted, blood is seen to be running behind the palate from the nasopharynx.

Traditionally a *gauze postnasal pack* is inserted. A catheter is passed along the anaesthetised nose until it appears behind the palate where it is grasped with forceps and pulled out of the mouth. A gauze pack sewn to tapes is then attached to the catheter by one of the tapes and, by pulling on the catheter, the pack is drawn into the postnasal space. The other tape comes from the mouth to enable the pack to be removed.

This is an unpleasant procedure, and children will almost always need a general anaesthetic, although some adults will tolerate the procedure without.

An easier way of controlling postnasal bleeding is the use of a *bladder catheter* with a 30 cc balloon. The lubricated catheter is inserted into the nose until the balloon is in the nasopharynx, where it is inflated. This procedure can be carried out without a general anaesthetic, even in a child, and is therefore of value in the control of post-adenoidectomy bleeding.

If the patient is elderly, or if the bleeding has been severe, admission to hospital will be appropriate. Nasal packing will then be removed after 24–48 hours.

If the bleeding recurs after removal of the pack the nose will be *repacked* and if, after a further 48 hours, the bleeding again recurs on removal of the pack, the patient will be taken to *the operating theatre* and the nose carefully *examined under general anaesthetic.* If the bleeding point can be seen it will be cauterised; if not the nose will be carefully packed.

If the bleeding recurs again then *arterial ligation* may be indicated. In cases of post-traumatic nose bleed, or if the bleeding is seen to be coming from the top of the nose, the *anterior ethmoidal artery* will be ligated. This artery is approached via a curved incision beneath the medial end of the eyebrow. A sub-periosteal dissection is carried out, and the artery will be seen running from the orbital contents to the lateral wall of the nose; it is controlled by diathermy clip or ligature.

If the bleeding is seen to be coming from the lower half of the nose the *maxillary artery* will be ligated.

The anterior wall of the maxillary sinus is opened via a sub-labial approach and the bone of the posterior wall gently broken and removed to expose the periosteum which covers the pterygo-palatine fossa. The pulsations of the maxillary artery can be seen through the periosteum and the artery is exposed and controlled by clip or ligature.

In severe bleeds the *external carotid artery* may be ligated, always above the first branch, to be certain that the correct artery is ligated, as the internal carotid has no branches. However, this artery is usually tied for bleeding which *cannot be controlled by packing*.

Investigations

In all patients the *blood pressure* will be measured, and in persistent or severe nose bleeds, a full blood count and clotting investigations will be performed and a *sinus X-ray* should be performed to exclude infection as a cause of the bleeding. However, after a severe bleed, opacity of the antrum may be caused by blood in the sinus.

Recurrent nose bleeds

In children the nose usually bleeds from Little's area as a result of moderate nasal trauma and infection of the nasal vestibule and prominent vessels may be cauterised. Five per cent cocaine is sprayed into the nose as a test dose, and a pledget of cotton wool soaked in 5 per cent cocaine but fully wrung out is inserted into the nose and left for 5–10 minutes. The vessels, which are then more prominent against the blanched mucosa, are cauterised by a silver nitrate stick held against the vessel for not less than 10–20 seconds. This technique is painless, and with careful management it is possible to carry it out in young children.

Other chemicals, including trichloracetic acid and chromic acid, or electric cautery may be used, but these are rather more harsh to the patient and to the nasal mucosa.

Both sides of the septum should not be cauterised at the same time, to avoid causing a perforation of the nasal septum.

Nasal Injuries

If seen immediately, there will be little swelling, and as the nose will still be numb from the injury it may be possible to correct an external deformity by firm pressure with the thumbs.

When seen some hours later in the surgery or casualty department, significant oedema is almost always present, and manipulation will be inappropriate. Three problems may be present at this time which will need urgent management.

1 Bleeding – see section on nose bleed.

2 Leak of cerebrospinal fluid (sugar present on urine testing stick) – these patients will need full neurosurgical evaluation.

3 Septal haematoma. After trauma bleeding occurs between the layers of the nasal septum, and the haematoma forms between the cartilage and the perichondrium. This devitalises the cartilage but, more seriously, this haematoma almost inevitably becomes infected, with the formation of a septal abscess which leads to dissolution of the septal cartilage with collapse of the nasal bridge.

Symptoms

1 Severe bilateral nasal obstruction.

2 Pain in the nose.

Signs

Septum red and swollen and soft to the probe.

Treatment

Under local or general anaesthetic the mucoperichondrium is incised on both sides of the septum and the haematoma is evacuated. Bilateral nasal packs are inserted to pack the mucoperichondrium against the cartilage, and antibiotics must be given for at least 1 week.

In the absence of a complication which necessitates urgent referral, a patient should be seen in an ENT clinic 7–10 days after a significant injury, which has caused either external deformity or nasal obstruction.

When seen the patient will be asked if the injury has changed the shape of his nose and, if so, the patient will be advised that to correct the deformity the nose must be manipulated within 2 weeks of the injury before the bones have 'set'.

If the nasal airway has been reduced by an acute deviation of the nasal septum, this can also be manipulated, but this procedure is less successful than manipulation for external deformity, as the septum tends to spring back into the abnormal position. Many of these patients will require a submucous resection of the nasal septum to correct the deformity.

Fractures of the middle third of the face

These fractures present complex problems which will be managed in a hospital either by the ENT department or by the facio-maxillary/oral surgeon. Details of these fractures and their management are not appropriate to this volume.

CHAPTER 3

THROAT

Examination

The light from an electric auriscope will suffice with a wooden tongue depressor. Two depressors will be needed to examine adequately the buccal mucosa between the teeth and cheeks and to view the sulcus between the side of the tongue and the tonsil, known as 'coffin corner', which is notorious for hiding small 'occult' tumours.

Lesions of the mouth should always be palpated to assess the texture and to determine if there is any surrounding induration or fixation. It is of great diagnostic importance to feel the posterior third of the tongue, as malignant lesions in this site may be totally invisible even on direct examination under anaesthetic, but can be felt as a hard lump.

Sore Throat

Viral pharyngitis

This is most often an uncomfortable but mild sore

throat which accompanies a viral upper respiratory tract infection. Symptomatic treatment is all that is required, and in the majority of cases antibiotics should not be given unless there is bacterial secondary infection.

Bacterial pharyngitis

This is caused by the infected postnasal discharge from chronic maxillary sinusitis running down the posterior pharyngeal wall.

Symptoms

1 Postnasal drip.

2 Persistent sore throat.

Signs

1 Mucopus in postnasal space which may be visible behind the soft palate when the patient gags.

2 Prominent inflamed lymphoid follicles on the posterior pharyngeal wall.

Investigation

Sinus X-ray will show opaque maxillary antra.

Treatment

The chronic infection of the maxillary antra should be treated as described in the section on sinusitis. On occasions the lymphoid follicles do not resolve completely, and they may be ablated by either cryotherapy or the carbon dioxide laser.

Acute tonsillitis

A severe sore throat with pyrexia, enlarged neck glands, focal exudate on the tonsils and malaise which is sufficiently severe to keep the child off school or the adult away from work.

Treatment with antibiotics is appropriate and, if the patient has had more than four attacks of acute tonsillitis per year for several years, tonsillectomy will be of value. However, the patient must be allowed to decide if he prefers the attacks of tonsillitis to the operation.

Quinsy

A peritonsillar abscess follows an attack of acute tonsillitis and the infection spreads to the plane between the tonsil and the superior constrictor muscle of the pharynx. The cellulitis develops into an abscess which pushes the tonsil, on the affected side, towards the mid-line.

Symptoms

1 Increasing pain on the affected side, often referred to the ear.

2 Trismus (an inability to open mouth).

3 Dysphagia.

Signs

1 Peritonsillar swelling.

2 Excessive salivation with drooling.

3 Trismus.

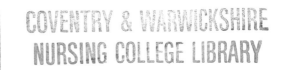

4 Palpable neck glands.

Treatment

1 If only cellulitis is present, antibiotics may be effective.

2 If pus has formed it must be drained.
   (a) Patient seated.
   (b) Local anaesthetic painted or sprayed onto most prominent point of abscess. Some believe that this is of no value to the patient as the tissues are so tightly stretched, but it at least has the advantage of persuading the patient that the throat has been anaesthetised, and he will then open his mouth for the abscess to be drained.
   (c) A guarded scalpel or quinsy forceps are used to open the abscess and this opening is then widened to allow drainage of the pus with immediate relief of pain.
   (d) Antibiotics should be given for 7 days.
   (e) A patient who has had a quinsy is likely to get another one, and tonsillectomy will be advised.

Glandular fever

Infective mononucleosis may present with a sore throat with marked enlargement of the neck glands. Classically there is a diffuse white exudate on the tonsils and petechial haemorrhages at the junction of the hard and soft palates. Diagnosis is confirmed by appropriate blood tests.

Treatment should be symptomatic and the course of the disease may be prolonged. Steroids may be of benefit in severe cases.

Scenario 2.

A client suffering from anorexia has been off
know if there is any evidence that such an ac
and self-confidence.

Question:	
	Keywords
P – Patient/Problem/ Population	
I - Intervention	
C - Comparison	
O- Outcome	

Thrush

A fungal infection with *Candida albicans* of the mouth and/or throat, with soreness and a white/yellow exudate which may look 'follicular'. Treatment is with an oral antifungal such as nystatin.

Dry throat from mouth-breathing

Inspired air is warmed and moistened by the nasal mucous membrane and if a patient does not breathe adequately through his nose, he inspires air which is excessively dry and cold. This results in a drying of the mucous membranes of the mouth and throat with minor atrophic changes, and the patient will complain of a persistent sore throat, which is often worse in the mornings after a night of mouth-breathing.

Abnormal signs in the throat in these cases are minimal, but an obvious cause for the nasal obstruction will usually be found and, when corrected, the sore throat usually resolves.

In addition, if abnormal occlusion of the teeth is present, this may prevent an individual from closing the mouth adequately, and these patients will inevitably mouth-breathe.

Dysphagia

Difficulty in swallowing is a cardinal symptom and all cases must be investigated by barium swallow and oesophagoscopy.

This section does not consider those painful conditions of the throat which cause the patient to be unwilling to swallow, but only those conditions in which the patient has actual difficulty in swallowing solids or liquids.

Dysphagia for solids indicates an obstructive lesion of the oesophagus, whereas dysphagia for liquids occurs in neurological disorders which may be either central or peripheral. The weakened muscles of the pharynx have more difficulty with the liquid than with a solid bolus of food, and in addition there is more tendency for liquids to spill over into the airway.

All cases of dysphagia must have a barium swallow, which is extremely accurate in showing up lesions between the cricopharyngeus and the stomach. However, small lesions may be present in the region of the cricopharyngeus muscle and in the food channels lateral to the larynx (the pyriform fossae), which do not show up well in a barium swallow. All patients must therefore have oesophagoscopy with a careful examination of the pharynx, pyriform fossae and post-cricoid region.

Oesophageal sensation is inaccurate, and obstruction at any site is frequently felt as a blockage in the suprasternal region.

Causes of dysphagia

Congenital

Atresia

This may occur with or without a tracheo-oesophageal fistula and, if gas is seen to be present in the stomach on X-ray, a fistula must be present between the trachea and the lower oesophageal segment. Complete dysphagia will be evident soon after birth, and it will not be possible to pass a nasogastric tube.

Treatment is by reconstruction by the paediatric/ thoracic surgical team when the child is fit.

Foreign body

A wide range of items are swallowed and become impacted in the oesophagus, including coins, false teeth, meat and fish bones, etc. The majority will stick in the cricopharyngeus region at the back of the larynx, which is the narrowest part of the gastro-intestinal tract, but obviously sharp objects may stick into the oesophageal wall at any level.

Symptoms

Sudden onset of severe dysphagia with pain in the throat during a meal.

Signs

1 Tenderness of the neck in the post-cricoid area.

2 Pain on moving the larynx from side to side.

3 If oedema has developed there will be loss of laryngeal crepitus – the grating of the larynx on the vertebrae which occurs when the larynx is moved from side to side.

4 Pooling of saliva in the pharynx visible with or without a mirror.

5 If perforation has occurred, surgical emphysema will be present – a crackling sensation in the subcutaneous tissues of the neck.

Investigation

Lateral X-ray of the neck to show the foreign body and, on occasions, a piece of cotton wool soaked in barium or a barium swallow may be needed.

Treatment

Removal of the foreign body under a general anaesthetic with full muscle relaxation.

Complications of a swallowed foreign body

Rupture of the oesophagus

This may occur when the bone is swallowed or when it is removed surgically.

The danger is that saliva will leak through the tear in the oesophagus and form a retropharyngeal abscess. This infection will then track down through the tissue planes of the neck into the mediastinum causing mediastinitis, which is still a dangerous and potentially lethal condition.

Symptoms

The symptoms will occur some time after oesophagoscopy and signs of rupture should have been identified before symptoms develop.

    1 Pain in neck.

    2 Dysphagia.

    3 Swelling of neck.

Signs

    1 Increased pulse.

2 Raised temperature.

3 Tenderness and swelling of neck.

4 Surgical emphysema.

Investigations

All patients who have been oesophagoscoped for foreign bodies and for other indications, should have a lateral X-ray of the neck and a chest X-ray performed to identify a leak which will be shown by the presence of air in the tissues. Air visible on X-ray may not be clinically detectable as surgical emphysema. The patient should not be permitted to swallow liquids until the X-rays have been performed and have shown to be normal.

Treatment

If the rupture appears to be very small and the patient's symptoms and signs are minimal, conservative treatment may be carried out.

1 Passage of nasogastric tube.

2 Nil by mouth.

3 Antibiotics.

However, the patient must be watched very carefully and if the condition deteriorates, or if the rupture appears to be large from the outset, the neck must be drained to prevent mediastinitis.

Drainage of the retropharyngeal area is carried out via an incision in the neck at the lower end of the sternomastoid muscle. Blunt dissection is used to enter the retro/para-oesophageal area where foul-smelling pus will be found. A drain will be inserted and

antibiotics given until X-ray with a non-irritant con-
strast medium shows that the tear has healed.

Small foreign bodies such as fish bones may stick in
the tonsils, base of tongue, valleculae – between the
tongue and epiglottis – and in the pyriform fossae.
Some can be removed with curved forceps under local
anaesthetic, but others may need a general anaesthetic.

Ingested corrosives

Aetiology

Suicide attempt or accident.

Symptoms

These depend on the severity of the oesophageal burn –
pain and dysphagia.

Signs

Burns of lips, mouth and throat.

Investigation

Determine nature of corrosive – look at label or call a
regional poisons unit which in the UK is at Guy's
Hospital.
   Oesophagoscopy should be performed to assess the
extent of oesophageal damage but not until the
patient's state is stable.

Treatment

   1 Dilute corrosive with water and aspirate the

stomach via wide tube. Do not make the patient vomit as this simply burns the oesophagus twice. Neutralisation of acid with alkali, and vice-versa, is dangerous and can produce gas.

2 Restore acid/base balance in the blood.

3 Prevent stricture formation by leaving a wide-bore nasogastric tube *in situ* and by the administeration of steroids. Antibiotics may have to be given to prevent secondary infection. If a stricture forms, repeated oesophagoscopy and dilatation will be needed.

Inflammation — reflux oesophagitis

Aetiology

Sliding hiatus hernia with reflux of gastric acid.

Symptoms

Heartburn, water brash, late stricture formation with dysphagia. Stricture formation is not common.

Signs

Nil.

Investigation

Barium swallow and oesophagoscopy.

Treatment

The patient is given intense medical treatment for his hiatus hernia and acid reflux and dilatation of the stricture will then be performed. If this is unsuccessful, and the stricture re-forms, surgical treatment of the hiatus hernia may be necessary, and this will be accompanied by further dilatation of the stricture.

Tumours

Benign – these tumours are rare and diagnosis will be made on barium swallow and oesophagoscopy with biopsy;

Malignant.

Aetiology

Smoking, spirit drinking, diet of spiced food, etc. Carcinoma from these causes is commoner in men in the lower two-thirds of the oesophagus, but in the upper one-third, carcinoma in women may be preceded by the Paterson, Brown-Kelly (Plummer Vinson) syndrome with iron deficiency anaemia. Other signs are koilonychia (spoon-shaped nails), smooth red tongue, angular stomatitis and a post-cricoid web, which is a small shelf in the upper oesophagus and is premalignant. Treatment of this premalignant condition is both by systemic iron and by dilatation of the stricture. In some cases the haemoglobin level may be normal, but the serum iron level may be low, and it should always be estimated.

Symptoms

Rapidly progressive dysphagia with weight loss. In upper third lesions there may be a preceding mild dysphagia from the Paterson, Brown-Kelly syndrome and there may also be voice changes from laryngeal involvement.

Signs

Obvious weight loss. Pooling of saliva in pyriform fossae visible on mirror laryngoscopy. Neck glands may be enlarged.

Investigation

Barium swallow – this will show the characteristic 'rat-tail' deformity. Oesophagoscopy with biopsy and histology almost always show squamous carcinoma but at the lower end there may be invasion by gastric carcinoma.

Treatment

Treatment of carcinoma of the middle and lower thirds of the oesophagus is carried out by general/thoracic surgeons. Treatment is by radiotherapy and/or surgery, and if this treatment fails then palliation may be achieved by inserting a plastic tube, endoscopically through the malignant stricture, enabling the patient to swallow his own saliva and a fluid diet.

Treatment of carcinoma of the upper third of the oesophagus is usually first by radiotherapy but, if this fails, then palliation with a tube is not possible as it cannot be tolerated behind the larynx. Whether or not to operate on these patients poses one of the most difficult problems in head and neck surgery. If the patient is fit and accepts surgery, two aims must be achieved. First, the patient should remain in hospital for as short a time as possible. Second, the patient's major symptom of dysphagia must be relieved. A high proportion (more than 80 per cent) of these patients will be dead within 2 years and they must have the quality of their life improved and must spend as little of it as possible in hospital.

The surgical excision is standard, a pharyngolaryngectomy, and the trachea is brought out through the skin of the neck as in a laryngectomy. The pharyngeal reconstruction may be carried out in several ways:

1 Plastic Stuart tube – only in non-irradiated cases.

2 Stomach pull-up – after mobilisation of the stomach the oesophagus and stomach are pulled up through the chest and the fundus of the stomach is anastomosed to the back of the pharynx.

3 Colon transplant – the right colon on its vascular pedicle is brought up and the caecum is joined to the pharynx and the ascending colon to the stomach. The oesophageal stump is sewn over.

4 Free graft of small bowel with microvascular anastomosis.

5 One-stage skin tube replacement using a medially-based chest flap.

Almost all cases have been irradiated and the operations of stomach pull-up, colon transplant and free graft of small bowel all involve two major operative sites. The use of a skin tube appears to offer slightly better results, possibly based on the fact that it is less shocking to the patient and therefore reduces his immune status less than the other procedures. However, it cannot be used in patients where the tumour descends significantly into the oesophagus, as when the oesophagus is divided low in the neck there is insufficient to anastomose to the side of the skin tube.

Neurological

Central

1 *Bulbar palsy* – any lesion of the brainstem which causes damage to the vagal nuclei will have dysphagia as one of its symptoms. If the dysphagia is severe, and if a barium swallow shows a significant hold-up at the level of the cricopharyngeus muscle, then a cricopharyngeal myotomy may be of benefit.

2 *Pseudobulbar palsy* – a similar symptomatology may be caused by an upper motor neuron lesion above the bulbar nuclei.

Peripheral

Pharyngeal pouch (Figure 3.1)

Aetiology

Neuromuscular incoordination between contraction of the pharynx and relaxation of the cricopharyngeal sphincter. A rise in intrapharyngeal pressure causes

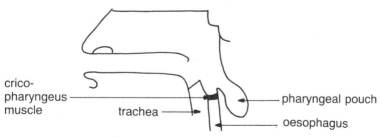

Figure 3.1   Pharyngeal pouch

mucosa of the pharynx to balloon out through a muscular weakness of the posterior pharyngeal wall – Killian's dehiscence.

Symptoms

Dysphagia, regurgitation of undigested food, a gurgling noise on swallowing as air is displaced from the pouch, cough and pneumonia from over-spill of fluid into the trachea and lump in the neck after swallowing – usually on the left side.

Investigation

Barium swallow and oesophagoscopy, which must always be performed to exclude a carcinoma within the pouch as these develop not infrequently.

Treatment

1 Excision of the pouch via an external incision with over-sewing of the defect and division of the cricopharyngeus muscle down to the mucosa to prevent a recurrence.

2 The Dohlman operation – if the patient is not fit the 'party wall' between the pouch and the oesophagus may be divided after diathermy using a special oesophagoscope (Figure 3.2). The party wall may be divided by the carbon dioxide laser.

Achalasia of the cardia

Aetiology

A failure of relaxation of the cardiac sphincter due to

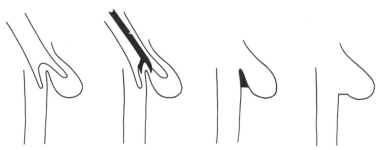

Figure 3.2 Treatment of a pharyngeal pouch by Dohlman's technique

degeneration of the nervous plexuses in the wall of the oesophagus.

Symptoms

Dysphagia and regurgitation.

Investigation

Diagnosis confirmed by barium swallow which shows a widely dilated oesophagus; oesophagoscopy will then be performed.

Treatment

Dilatation of the sphincter with mercury-filled bougies or Heller's operation in which the cardiac sphincter muscle is divided down to mucosa.

Diffuse oesophageal spasm

In this condition uncoordinated swallowing with spasm forces the bolus up and down the oesophagus causing significant discomfort.

Symptoms

Pain and dysphagia.

Investigation

Barium swallow.

Treatment

Muscle relaxant therapy and, if this fails, division of the circular muscle of the oesophagus from cricopharyngeus to cardia may be necessary.

Globus hystericus

Aetiology

Probably psychosomatic.

Symptoms

A sensation of a lump in the throat but *no* dysphagia.

Signs

None.

Treatment

The patient may be told that he has a patch of muscle spasm in the throat which is causing the sensation of a lump, and that this causes him to worry, thus increasing the spasm and the sensation. Patients must be reassured strongly that there is no organic disease and given diazepan to 'relax the muscle spasm'. The majority of patients will respond to this regime but in those patients whose symptoms persist, many will require barium swallow and oesophagoscopy.

This diagnosis cannot be made if there is any true dysphagia.

The Larynx

Stridor

Inspiratory stridor indicates upper respiratory tract obstruction, and it is a symptom which must be investigated as a matter of extreme urgency.

Hoarseness

This is also a most important cardinal symptom and the larynx must be examined in all patients who have persistent hoarseness for 4–6 weeks. If it is not possible to examine the larynx perfectly, in the clinic with a mirror, then the examination must be carried out under a general anaesthetic and, of course, lesions seen with a mirror will be examined and biopsied under anaesthetic.

Persistent hoarseness may be caused by an organic lesion in the larynx, or by damage to one of the recurrent laryngeal nerves.

Laryngoscopy

Mirror laryngoscopy is not easy to perform and, in many patients, experts cannot get an adequate view of the larynx even after spraying the throat with local anaesthetic.

If a practitioner is not performing mirror laryngoscopy regularly, it is difficult to perform it adequately, and lesions may be missed.

It is probably wise to refer urgently every patient with persistent hoarseness to an ENT clinic for laryngoscopy to make an early diagnosis, and to be certain that small and potentially curable malignant lesions are not missed.

Laryngeal disease

Some laryngeal disorders present with hoarseness and, as the disease process advances, stridor may develop. However, other disorders will present with acute stridor.

Congenital

Webs

A web may be present between the vocal cords and the symptoms will vary from hoarseness to obstruction with stridor. An airway may be created by perforating the web surgically, but complete removal of the web is difficult. Even after division with the carbon dioxide laser an indwelling stent may be needed for several weeks to prevent reformation of the web.

Cysts

These are rare and the symptoms will depend on the

size. Surgical treatment is relatively easy and should be successful.

Subglottic stenosis

This is a congenital narrowing of the airway at the level of the cricoid cartilage below the vocal cords. If the narrowing is not too severe it may present during the child's first upper respiratory tract infection and an urgent tracheostomy may be needed.

If after the infection has resolved the child cannot be decannulated, one of two treatment methods is available:

1 Conservative – the tracheostomy tube is left *in situ* for up to 2 years until decannulation can be achieved. During this time a speaking valve must be attached to the tracheostomy tube, which is fenestrated at the angle so that air can be inspired through the tube and expired through the larynx. This passage of air through the larynx is essential to 'dilate' the larynx, which will then grow normally.

2 Surgical – the operation of laryngo-tracheoplasty – the larynx is opened anteriorly via a longitudinal incision, the stenotic area is cut back and the circumference of the cricoid cartilage enlarged by the placement of a cartilage graft in the anterior incision.

Trauma to the recurrent laryngeal nerves

This may occur during delivery and is almost always unilateral. The hoarseness caused by unilateral vocal cord paralysis may be permanent.

Trauma

Voice misuse

1 *Acute* – patients who misuse their voice may develop a submucosal haematoma of the vocal cords.

   If a patient continues to use his voice during an attack of acute laryngitis, further oedema may develop which will prolong the period of hoarseness and may eventually lead to chronic laryngitis. Patients with acute laryngitis must be advised to rest the voice, to stop smoking, and to use inhalations. Antibiotics may be prescribed.

2 *Chronic* – the patient is often a teacher or someone who has to use his voice in a noisy or polluted environment. The voice quality tends to deteriorate towards the end of the day.

This is not really a pathological situation but the normal response of the larynx to an abnormal situation. The patient must be advised accordingly that there is no medical disorder or specific treatment for this condition. Training in voice production and speech therapy may help, and during an acute attack voice rest is essential.

Chronic voice misuse may cause the patient to develop singer's nodes, known as screamer's nodes in children. As a result of repeated violent adductions of the vocal cords, firm fibrous nodules develop at the junction of the anterior one-third and posterior two-thirds of the vocal cords. Early lesions may resolve with speech therapy, but if this fails, surgical removal, either by forceps or the carbon dioxide laser may be necessary. This will be followed by speech therapy to prevent recurrence.

External trauma

A sharp lacerating or penetrating injury is easy to diagnose, but may pose many difficult problems in management and reconstruction.

Blunt trauma poses problems in both diagnosis and management. The diagnosis is often missed as laryngeal trauma commonly occurs in a patient with multiple injuries who requires intubation for ventilation. Once this has been performed, the larynx tends to be forgotten.

Symptoms

From hoarseness to obstruction with stridor.

Signs

Evidence of neck injury. The larynx is tender and surgical emphysema may be present in the neck.

Investigation

Mirror laryngoscopy and neck X-rays. Direct laryngoscopy with or without tracheostomy and surgical exploration of the neck may be necessary.

Treatment

Patients with oedema or small haematomas should be observed and steroids may, on occasions, be given.

If a severe injury has occurred with fracture of the laryngeal cartilages, the neck must be explored with removal of devitalised cartilage fragments and wiring of major fragments. In addition, lacerations of the mucosa are repaired and then a soft indwelling prosthesis must be inserted into the larynx to prevent stenosis. This prosthesis should be left *in situ* for 6–8 weeks.

Prolonged endotracheal intubation

It is difficult to define prolonged endotracheal intubation but, from a number of series, the incidence of stenosis appears to be of the order of 17–20 per cent.

The maximum safe period for intubation still remains uncertain and appears to vary with the age of the patient. There is evidence to suggest that a tube may be left longer in a small child than in an adult.

However, with all patients a decision should be made after approximately 72 hours of endotracheal intubation. If it appears certain that the tube can be removed within a further 3–5 days, then the tube may be left *in situ*. If not, then the tube should be changed for a tracheostomy.

The stenosis which follows prolonged intubation occurs from damage by the tube to the airway at the cricoid ring, and stenosis at this level poses immense problems, particularly if perichondritis with collapse of the cartilage occurs.

Post-intubation granuloma

This occurs after a prolonged anaesthetic from the irritative effects of the anaesthetic tube lying in the posterior part of the space between the vocal cords. Diagnosis is made on the history, and the finding of a pink granuloma arising from one arytenoid cartilage at the posterior part of the larynx.

Treatment is by removal of the granuloma followed by either the injection of steroids or systemic steroids. Even after this treatment, recurrence is not uncommon.

Foreign bodies

The site at which a foreign body becomes impacted depends upon its size and whether it is caught in the larynx by spasm. Relief of the acute obstruction may be possible on occasions by holding the patient (usually a child) upside-down and violently compressing the chest to expel the foreign body. A cricothyrotomy or tracheostomy may be performed if it is possible to get below the obstruction.

Removal of a foreign body which is not completely occluding the airway is a difficult procedure and poses both anaesthetic and surgical problems.

Inhaled peanuts break up in the lungs with the release of peanut oil which causes inflammation and a lung abscess.

Burns

Any patient who has sustained a burn to the airway is in grave danger of developing severe laryngeal oedema which may form rapidly some hours after the burn. Any patient who has evidence of a burn around the mouth, or particularly in the mouth or throat, must be kept under very careful observation.

Some polystyrene ceiling tiles melt in a fire, filling the air with polystyrene vapour which is inhaled and then resolidifies in the lungs, causing severe respiratory problems.

Inflammation

Acute

Acute Laryngitis

Aetiology

Viral during an upper respiratory tract infection with bacterial supra-infection.

Symptoms

Malaise, discomfort in throat and hoarseness.

Investigation

Mirror laryngoscopy will show red oedematous vocal cords.

Treatment

The patient must be advised to rest his voice, to give up smoking and to use inhalations. Antibiotics may be prescribed in severe cases.

Croup

Aetiology

Known as acute laryngo-tracheo-bronchitis. It is a more diffuse inflammatory process throughout the whole of the airway.

Symptoms

Malaise, cough, hoarseness with the development of

upper airway obstruction with dyspnoea and stridor.

Signs

A sick, distressed child with pyrexia and dyspnoea with stridor.

Investigation and treatment

See acute epiglottitis.

Acute epiglottitis

Aetiology

Infection of the epiglottis by *Haemophilus influenza*. Oedema and airway obstruction develop rapidly.

Symptoms

Rapid onset of hoarseness, dyspnoea and stridor during an otherwise relatively trivial upper respiratory tract infection.

Signs

A very ill, distressed child with dyspnoea and stridor.

Investigation

All investigations and examinations of the child must be carried out extremely carefully and only when facilities are available for the relief of complete respiratory obstruction. It has been reported that a number of relatively minor examinations and investigations, such as examining the mouth with a tongue depressor, and venepuncture, have caused complete respiratory obstruction.

Each child must be managed on merit in the knowledge that complete obstruction may develop suddenly without warning and with potentially fatal consequences.

On examination of the mouth, the epiglottis may be seen to be red and swollen behind the tongue, and a lateral X-ray of the neck shows soft tissue swelling of the epiglottis.

Treatment

Children with acute epiglottitis, which cannot necessarily be distinguished from a severe attack of croup, must be kept under constant and vigilant observation. Conservative treatment should be given.

1 Antibiotics (the antibiotic must be effective against *Haemophilus influenzae*).

2 Steriods.

3 Humidification.

4 Mild sedation may, on occasions, be given with great care.

If the respiratory obstruction does not improve rapidly, of if there is any evidence of severe deterioration, then either endotracheal intubation or tracheostomy must be performed. The choice between these two measures depends on the personnel available, but assuming that both high-quality anaesthetic and ENT staff are available, then intubation would now appear to be the treatment of choice as it has a significantly lower morbidity. However, if intubation is unsuccessful the tube may provoke spasm with complete respiratory obstruction and intubation must never be attempted unless an experienced surgeon is present to carry out an urgent tracheostomy if this occurs.

It is often difficult to distinguish a severe attack of croup from acute epiglottitis, although the history of the rapidity of the development of obstruction may aid the diagnosis. All cases with obstruction and stridor must be treated as a matter of extreme urgency.

Diphtheria

This is now extremely rare but, in the past, obstruction was caused by a dirty, grey-white membrane which could not be wiped or sucked off the mucosa of the throat and larynx.

Chronic inflammation

Chronic laryngitis

Aetiology

Failure to treat acute laryngitis correctly – usually the patient cannot rest his voice or stop smoking.

Smoking, chest infection, chronic sinus infection and voice misuse.

Oedema of the vocal cord mucosa develops which may be generalised or localised in the form of polyps.

Symptoms

Hoarseness, which may at first be intermittent, with the voice returning to normal between attacks. However, the hoarseness eventually becomes persistent and other symptoms will be related to the cause of the laryngitis; namely, cough, postnasal discharge, etc.

Investigation

Laryngoscopy, sinus X-ray and chest X-ray.

Treatment

Any underlying cause should be treated, if possible. At laryngoscopy the oedematous mucosa may be stripped and polypi removed, either with micro-instruments or with the carbon dioxide laser.

Tumours

Benign

A wide range of benign tumours can occur in the larynx with symptoms of voice change and/or obstruction. However, significant benign tumours are rare.

Recurrent respiratory papillomatosis

An uncommon, benign tumour which causes serious problems, particularly in children, is viral laryngeal papillomatosis. In this condition the larynx becomes filled with frond-like viral warts with symptoms of hoarseness and laryngeal obstruction with stridor. The risk of obstruction is obviously greatest when the larynx is small.

Aetiology

These viral papillomata may occasionally be found in children of mothers with genital warts.

Pathology

The disease often presents between the ages of 2 and 5 years and in the past it was thought that a majority of cases would remit at about the time of puberty. In the past it was known as juvenile laryngeal papillomatosis, but now many think that it should be called recurrent respiratory papillomatosis as, not infrequently, the disease continues into adult life. A wide range of techniques has been used to remove the papillomata, but to date no reliable method has been found to prevent recurrence, which may be at intervals of weeks or even days.

Symptoms

Hoarseness and airway obstruction with stridor.

Treatment

The aim of any surgical removal must be to remove the papillomata without causing damage to the normal larynx, which would cause scarring and stenosis.

Children in whom recurrence is rapid require scores of procedures to preserve the airway, and within the last few years it has become evident that using the carbon dioxide surgical laser it is possible to perform precise, bloodless removal of all the papillomata without the nuisance bleeding which other techniques provoke and with minimal damage to normal laryngeal tissues. In the post-operative period there is negligible oedema and a minimal chance of post-operative scarring and contracture.

Premalignant lesions

Leukoplakia may develop in the larynx as a result of chronic irritation. Possible irritants include smoking, poor dental hygiene, sinusitis, etc.

At laryngoscopy the lesion will be removed by excision biopsy under the operating microscope and histology will show one of the following:

1 Hyperkeratosis with normal cellular and cell layer architecture.

2 Hyperkeratosis with atypical cells or cellular architecture.

3 Carcinoma *in situ.*

4 Invasive carcinoma.

In the absence of invasive carcinoma, treatment should be by removal of any obvious irritant and by careful follow-up with removal for microscopy of any recurrent lesions.

Malignant

Aetiology

It would appear certain that carcinoma of the larynx is related to smoking.

Pathology

The larynx is divided into three parts: the glottis, the region around the vocal cords, and, above them, the supraglottic and, below, the subglottic regions. Glottic carcinoma is by far the most common, followed by supraglottic and, finally, subglottic lesions which are fortunately rare.

Symptoms

1 Glottic carcinoma – any lesion of the vocal cords, even when tiny, will present with hoarseness. This means that glottic carcinoma presents very early and, as there is poor lymphatic drainage from the vocal cords, its spread to lymph nodes in the neck is late.

2 Supraglottic – there is more space above the vocal cords for a tumour to develop without causing symptoms, and these tumours can develop to a significant size before presenting with a less well-defined gruffness of the voice. Spread to extra-laryngeal tissues may be accompanied by pain which is often referred to the ear. Spread to lymph nodes is relatively early.

3 Subglottic – these tumours can develop for a significant period of time without symptoms, and not infrequently they present with a sudden onset of respiratory obstruction with stridor, when over a period of a few days or even hours the size of the tumour produces a critical level of airway obstruction. Spread to lymph nodes is relatively early and spread within the lymph node chain proceeds downwards into the superior mediastinum when treatment becomes extremely difficult, if not impossible.

Signs

A hoarse voice, stridor with large tumours and subglottic tumours and enlarged lymph nodes in the neck.

Investigation

Laryngoscopy and biopsy. Histology almost invariably shows squamous carcinoma. Chest X-ray.

Treatment

In Britain the vast majority of cases will receive a full course of radiotherapy and surgery will be reserved for residual or recurrent tumours.

Immediate surgery may, on occasions, be carried out

on tumours which invade the laryngeal cartilages and on tumours which are large enough to cause respiratory obstruction when the alternative to an immediate laryngectomy is a tracheostomy, with its danger of seeding of tumour around the stoma. However, the introduction of the carbon dioxide laser has meant that obstructing tumours can be debulked with a temporary restoration of the airway, so that appropriate treatment can be planned at leisure.

A relatively small number of cases are suitable for a partial laryngectomy – either horizontal, in which the larynx above the vocal cords is removed, or vertical, in which one side of the larynx is excised.

However, in a majority of cases, if residual or recurrent tumour is present, a total laryngectomy will be performed. Although this is a relatively minor operation which is well tolerated by patients of all ages, it has the major sequel of loss of voice.

Oesophageal speech may be learnt by many patients, but a number will not be able to develop this skill and for these, vibrating electronic aids are available. A new development in speech rehabilitation is the introduction of valves between the trachea and oesophagus, and although many successes have been achieved they are not widely used, and spillover of saliva into the trachea appears to be a significant complication of their use.

Neurological

Vagal lesions

These may be either central, or the nerve may be involved by pathology at the base of the skull. In cases where the nerve is involved at a high level the palate on the affected side will be paralysed, and on gagging will rise towards the normal side. In addition, damage to the superior laryngeal nerve will affect the cricothyroid muscle on that side, and in addition to an immobile vocal cord there may be evidence of a reduction in tension in the vocal cord with bowing.

Recurrent laryngeal nerve lesions

The recurrent laryngeal nerve on the right side is the shorter of the two and it hooks around the subclavian artery. On the left side the nerve hooks around the ductus arteriosus in the superior mediastinum and both nerves then travel upwards to the larynx in the groove between the trachea and the oesophagus.

If the left vocal cord is paralysed it must be assumed that the patient has a carcinoma of the bronchus on the left side until proved otherwise.

Thyroid surgery

If one recurrent laryngeal nerve is cut it will give the typical abnormal voice with breathy hoarseness. The paralysed vocal cord lies in the paramedian position, just lateral to the midline, and the normal cord cannot adduct adequately to meet it, giving rise to escape of air with the classical voice abnormality. If recovery does not take place within 6 months, or if it is certain that the recurrent laryngeal nerve has been cut, then Teflon can be injected into the paralysed cord, causing it to swell to the midline so that the active cord can achieve vocal cord closure and a much more normal voice.

Bilateral recurrent laryngeal nerve palsy causes a life-threatening laryngeal obstruction with both vocal cords just lateral to the midline and a very small glottic chink. Some patients can lead a fairly normal life with this degree of obstruction but it tends to become very much worse during an upper respiratory tract infection.

Treatment of this condition is by moving one vocal cord laterally, and this may be done in Woodman's operation by placing a stitch round one cord to abduct it. More recently, endoscopic removal of the arytenoid cartilage and part of the vocal cord using the carbon dioxide laser appears to give consistently satisfactory results.

When both cords are in the paramedian position the voice is good. However, moving a cord laterally will improve the airway but cause the voice to deteriorate.

Unilateral recurrent laryngeal nerve paralysis

If the left side is affected as mentioned above, this must be diagnosed as carcinoma of the bronchus until proved otherwise. The patient submitted to X-rays, sputum cytology, bronchoscopy, etc. This nerve may also be affected by cardiac and aortic pathology. The right nerve may be affected by an apical carcinoma of the right lung.

Viral

Idiopathic recurrent laryngeal nerve paralysis is thought to be due to a virus but this is a diagnosis which can be made after serious pathology has been excluded.

Allergy

Allergic oedema of the larynx can be treated by

steroids or, if less severe, by antihistamines.

Rheumatoid arthritis

This disease may affect the joints between the cricoid and the arytenoid cartilages, fixing the vocal cords in a midline position. This causes airway obstruction and may, on occasions, require a tracheostomy with a speaking valve.

Congenital laryngeal stridor – laryngomalacia

This is by far the commonest cause of stridor in infants and is caused by a failure of stiffening of the laryngeal cartilages. On inspiration the excessively soft supraglottic structures are sucked into the glottis, causing stridor.

All children with stridor must be submitted to laryngoscopy to confirm the diagnosis, but when laryngomalacia has been diagnosed, the parents can be reassured that the child is not in any danger, and that the condition will improve as the child grows older and the cartilages stiffen.

Tracheostomy

The operation of tracheostomy is performed in a wide range of surgical and medical disciplines. If surgery and management are of a high standard the morbidity and incidence of complications are extremely low.

However, if surgery is imperfectly performed or management is poor, then significant and severe complications can occur.

Indications

1 To relieve upper airway obstruction.

2 To aspirate the tracheobronchial tree.

3 To protect the tracheobronchial tree from:
   (a) blood,
   (b) secretions.

4 In patients with respiratory failure:
   (a) to allow intermittent, positive pressure ventilation,
   (b) in cases of chronic failure to reduce the dead space.

5 To permit surgical access to mouth, pharynx and larynx.

6 After laryngectomy (not really a true tracheostomy).

To relieve upper airway obstruction

The causes of obstruction have been covered in the section on diseases of the larynx and obstruction may also occur in cases of severe trauma to the face and jaws. The urgency of the procedure will be determined by the severity of the obstruction.

To aspirate the tracheobronchial tree

This is necessary in cases of sputum retention in

patients who are either unable, or unwilling, to clear their lung secretions. This may occur after chest or abdominal surgery or injury and, in some cases, of debility. A vicious circle is set up from the initial retention of sputum:

1 Alveoli become filled with sputum →

2 Reduced pulmonary ventilation →

3 Accumulation of carbon dioxide →

4 Central depression with further reduction in tendency to cough →

5 Further accumulation of sputum →

6 A continuation of this vicious cycle to death.

Treatment

1 Prevention by physiotherapy, postural drainage, etc.

2 Once sputum retention has been established, bronchoscopy will be performed, usually without the need for anaesthetic to aspirate the tracheobronchial tree. After that physiotherapy will be given, to prevent a recurrence.

3 However, if recurrence occurs, then a tracheostomy may be necessary to allow repeated suction of the tracheobronchial tree which is extremely difficult via an endotracheal tube.

Protection of the tracheobronchial tree

Against blood

After major facial and jaw trauma or surgery there

may be a danger of aspiration of blood. A tracheostomy is frequently performed as a routine in major head and neck surgery to remove the danger of aspiration if reactionary or secondary haemorrhage occurs.

Against secretions

In the unconscious or paralysed patient, aspiration will normally be prevented by postural drainage and physiotherapy. However, on occasions – if the patient has had a major injury which prevents regular change in posture, such as a fractured femur, pelvis, spine or chest – then a tracheostomy may be needed to keep the lungs clear of secretions. A cuffed tube will be needed in these cases.

Respiratory failure

Acute

Many patients who require intermittent positive pressure ventilation will be managed initially with an endotracheal tube. However, if this has to be left *in situ* for more than 1 week it must be changed for a tracheostomy to avoid the danger of laryngeal stenosis at the level of the cricoid cartilage.

Chronic

A tracheostomy is rarely performed to improve pulmonary function by reducing the dead space by half.

Access

If surgery to the mouth, pharynx or larynx has to be performed, the presence of an endotracheal tube within the operative field will often make this extremely

difficult, if not impossible. In these cases a tracheostomy will be performed for surgical access.

After laryngectomy

This is not truly a tracheostomy but the trachea after
surgery is brought out as an end tracheostomy through
the skin of the neck.

The operation of tracheostomy

In an emergency it is preferable to insert a specially
designed trocar and cannula through the membrane
between the cricoid and thyroid cartilages. If this
cannula is not available then a wide-bore needle may
be used at this site or even into the trachea. This
temporary relief of the obstruction will allow time for
an elective tracheostomy to be performed at leisure.

Anaesthetic

For the performance of a tracheostomy the anaesthetic
used will depend on the urgency of the procedure. In a
dire emergency no anaesthetic will be used and, in
those cases where endotracheal intubation is not
possible but where there is no great hurry, then the
operation will be carried out under local anaesthetic. In
elective cases the ideal situation is to perform the
operation under general anaesthetic with an endotracheal tube *in situ*.

Position of the patient

The head is extended with a pillow under the shoulders. The patient must be positioned in a straight line on the table to ensure that the trachea is in the midline of the neck. The accurate alignment of the patient is not critically important in adults, where the trachea is readily palpable, but it is very important in children where the trachea is only a few millimetres in diameter and may be very difficult to find.

Incision

In an emergency a midline vertical incision is the most rapid but healing is with an unsightly midline scar which tends to contract. If the operation is less urgent then a horizontal skin crease 'thyroidectomy incision' heals with the best scar.

Operation

Once the incision has been made and skin flaps elevated, dissection is in the midline where a bloodless plane exists. Only the thyroid isthmus crosses this midline and this will be clamped and divided. Rarely, the innominate artery rises up in front of the trachea in children and must be looked for and avoided.

Trachea

In an adult a window must be cut in the anterior wall of the trachea, not higher than the second ring, and some prefer to turn down the flap of anterior tracheal wall and suture it to the skin as a Bjork flap to aid replacement of the tracheostomy tube. In a child the tracheal cartilages have not calcified and are very soft and flexible; here a vertical slit is made at a similar level and turned into a diamond-shaped opening using tracheal dilators.

The tube

An appropriately sized tube will be inserted. In a child the size of the trachea, and therefore the tube, is the same as the external diameter of the terminal phalanx of the child's little finger.

Plastic and metal tubes are available and plastic tubes may be both cuffed and uncuffed. The advantage of using a metal tube is that it has an inner tube which can be removed for cleaning, if it becomes blocked, without removing the outer tube from the neck. If a plastic tube becomes blocked then the whole tube must be removed for cleaning and it may sometimes be difficult to change tubes, particularly within a few hours of the operation.

A cuffed tube will be used for intermittent positive pressure ventilation and in cases where the tracheo-bronchial tree must be protected.

Tube fixation

If the tracheostomy tube is correctly tied in place it will not become displaced. When the neck is extended it has a greater circumference than when flexed, and if the tube is tied in place with the neck extended the tapes will become loose once the neck is flexed. Therefore it is vitally important to flex the neck before tying the tube tapes in place.

Tracheostomy care

Communication

The patient cannot talk and will need a bell, pencil and paper.

Humidification

The nose and mouth are no longer in the airway to warm and moisten the inspired air. If the inspired air is not humified, secretions will dry in the trachea and will gradually obstruct the airway. For the first 2 weeks full humidification of the tracheostome must be carried out, but after this time the trachea becomes accustomed to relatively dry air. A moist gauze square over the tracheostome will suffice for humidification.

New tube

A new tube of identical specifications, with tracheal dilators and a light, must be available by the bed of the patient to replace the tube if it becomes blocked.

Suction

This must be available to keep the tracheobronchial tree free from secretions. A full aseptic technique must be observed, and in order to achieve adequate suction the suction catheter must not be sucking when it is inserted into the trachea or it will become attached to the tracheal or the bronchial wall by suction. In this case a full insertion and adequate suction will not be possible. Suction must only be turned on as the catheter is withdrawn.

Problems and complications

Tube displacement

This will not be possible if the tube is tied in correctly with the neck flexed.

Tube blocked

Breathing through a tracheostomy is silent, and if
breathing can be heard it means that the tube is
narrowed by secretions on the walls, and that a
turbulent air flow with 'stridor' has developed. The
tube must be cleared immediately by suction and, if
this is unsuccessful, a plastic tube must be changed
completely or the inner tube of a metal tube should be
removed for cleaning.

Cuff problems

The inflated cuff can cause ischaemic damage to the
tracheal wall by vessel compression. It should be
deflated for 5 minutes each hour, or 10 minutes every 2
hours to avoid this problem. Some new low-pressure
cuffs or double cuffs are available to overcome this
problem. If tracheal stenosis is caused its treatment is
extremely difficult, and requires excision of the sten-
osed area with end-to-end anastomosis. This can only
be performed for relatively short lengths of trachea.

Infection

If this occurs the tracheostomy care has been imperfect.

Decannulation problems

Children find it extremely easy to breathe through a
tracheostomy and often find great difficulty in re-
establishing breathing through the normal airway.
Partial corking of the tracheostomy may aid decannulation but, on occasions, it is necessary to remove the

tracheostomy tube under anaesthetic and replace this with a naso-tracheal airway, which can be removed after a few days.

Stenosis

In addition to problems caused by the cuff, a portion of the anterior wall of the trachea can be pushed in by a tube which is too large for the window cut in the anterior wall.

Fistula into the oesophagus

This is rare and may be caused by a badly-angled metal tube eroding the posterior tracheal wall.

Tube too long

A long tube may enter the right main bronchus and fail to ventilate the left lung. This problem can be detected by X-ray and clinical observation.

After removal of the tube the stoma will heal without the need for suture. A persistent fistula is rare and can easily be repaired. On occasions the cosmetic appearance of a healed tracheostomy scar is unacceptable to the patient, and can be corrected by excision and scar revision.

CHAPTER 4

THE EARS

Examination

The pinna

This should be examined for surgical scars, particularly in the post-auricular sulcus. In cases of external otitis, swelling of the pinna will indicate the development of perichondritis, which requires urgent systemic antibiotic treatment.

External meatus

For examination the pinna should be gently pulled backwards straightening the meatus. Boils may occur in the hair-bearing outer part of the meatus. The presence or absence of wax or the discharge of otitis externa will be looked for. Wax will not form in an infected ear canal and its return, after an attack of otitis externa, is an encouraging sign.

The ear drum

The ear drum should appear like clear, translucent glass. (The author once saw a flower shop's plate-glass window with water running down the back of it, which looked exactly like the appearance of a normal ear drum.)

There is a light reflex in the antero-inferior quadrant but the key to the examination of the ear drum is the handle of the malleus, which remains intact even with enormous subtotal perforations of the pars tensa.

When the handle of the malleus has been identified the rest of the ear drum can be related to it.

It is wise to examine the normal ear first in unilateral disease, to determine the depth, angulation and anatomy of the normal drum. On occasions, it is possible to look through a large perforation without seeing the rim of ear drum and to think that the medial wall of the middle ear is in fact the drum, if the depth of the normal drum has not first been assessed.

Tests of Hearing

First the level of hearing in the two ears should be tested with the voice, and it is important to ensure that when one ear is being tested, the sound is not heard in the other. The non-tested ear should be masked to prevent this.

Test	*Masking*
Whisper	Finger in meatus
Conversation	Paper scratched over meatus
Shout	Barany noise box

Second, the hearing is tested with a tuning fork.

The Rinne test (Figure 4.1)

This test is carried out with a 512 Hz tuning fork. Air conduction of the vibrations of the tuning fork through the normal sound pathway is compared with bone conduction when the sound waves are transmitted from the bone of the mastoid process directly to the cochlea.

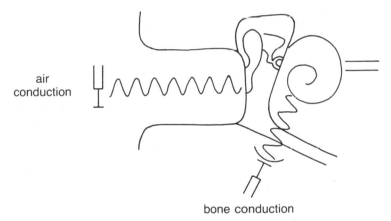

Figure 4.1   Rinne test.

The patient is asked which is louder.

Normal:	air conduction is better than bone conduction = Rinne positive
Sensorineural deafness:	air conduction is better than bone conduction = Rinne positive
Conductive deafness:	bone conduction is better than air conduction = Rinne negative (Figure 4.2).

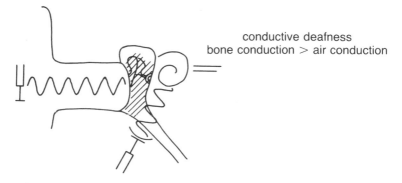

conductive deafness
bone conduction > air conduction

Figure 4.2   Rinne test – negative Rinne

In cases of severe unilateral sensorineural deafness, if the level of hearing has not first been assessed with the voice, when the tuning fork is presented to the meatus for air conduction it will not be heard, but when bone conduction is tested this will be present as the sound waves are conducted across the skull to the opposite cochlea. However, this may not be noticed by the patient. There will therefore appear to be a negative Rinne test, but this pitfall can be avoided if the hearing level is tested with the voice before the tuning fork tests are performed.

The Weber test (Figure 4.3)

In this test the tuning fork is placed on the forehead of the patient and sound waves travel through the bone equally to both cochleas. The patient is then asked in which ear the sound is louder. In unilateral sensorineural deafness the sound will obviously be heard in the better ear with the normal cochlea. However, in unilateral conductive deafness the sound will be heard in the deaf ear which is masked from external sounds

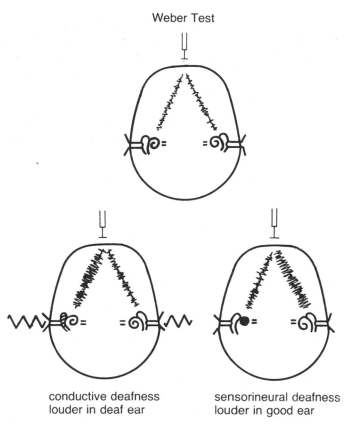

Weber Test

conductive deafness
louder in deaf ear

sensorineural deafness
louder in good ear

Figure 4.3   Weber test

by the conductive deafness and can therefore 'concentrate' better on the bone-conducted sounds.

Anatomy of the Middle Ear Air Spaces

The ear drum is the gateway to a system of spaces

within the temporal bone (Figure 4.4). These can only be reached surgically by removing the overlying bone at the operation of mastoidectomy.

Above the middle ear is a space called the attic, containing the head of the malleus and the body of the incus. This leads via a passage – the aditus – to the mastoid antrum which is connected to the foamy air cells which fill the mastoid process. The mastoid process is pulled from the side of the head by the sternomastoid muscle when the child first raises his head, and until this time the facial nerve emerges from the side of the head behind the ear and is significantly at risk in a post-auricular surgical incision. When the mastoid process has formed it protects the nerve from this danger.

Physiology

Sound waves are collected by the pinna, which can

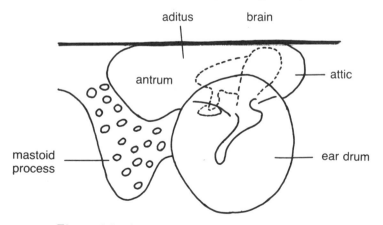

Figure 4.4   Anatomy of the middle ear air spaces

move in animals but not in man. However, we still have vestigial muscles behind the ear which contract when a sound is heard, and these contractions can be recorded electrically and used as a basis for an objective hearing test which does not demand the co-operation of the patient. These tests are of great value in children, disturbed adults and medico-legal cases.

Sound waves cause the ear drum to vibrate, and these vibrations are transmitted via the ossicular chain to the inner ear fluids, where the mechanical vibrations are changed into electrical impulses which are transmitted to the brain via the VIIIth nerve.

The 'middle ear structures' (Figure 4.5) magnify the sound eighteen times to overcome the problem of transmitting sound waves across an air/fluid interface at which a majority of the sound is reflected (this can be confirmed by placing one's head under water when

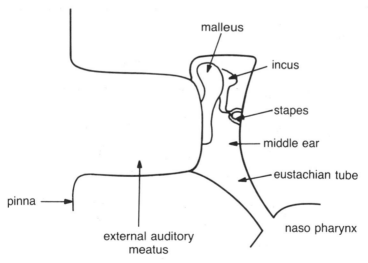

Figure 4.5 External and middle ear structures

someone is talking). The vibrations of the large drum are 'focused' onto the tiny stapes footplate and the ossicular chain acts as a lever system with a small mechanical advantage.

Cochlea

Within the inner ear the tuned basilar membrane is caused to vibrate by the sound waves, and these vibrations are identified with regards to pitch and volume by the organ of Corti.

Deafness

Deafness may be conductive when any part of the apparatus from external meatus to stapes footplate is abnormal, and perceptive when there is a disorder in the inner ear or VIIIth nerve. Perceptive deafness is now widely known as sensorineural with sensory deafness due to cochlear, and neural to VIIIth nerve, disease.

Vestibular apparatus

There are two parts to the vestibular apparatus – the organ of balance. First, the semicircular canals: movements of the head cause a movement of the fluid in the semicircular canals and these organs give information on the speed and direction of head movements. Second, the otolith organs: these are static position receptors. Within the 'jelly' which lies over the hair cells are otoliths (ear stones) and these fall by gravity onto the hair cells when the head is in a particular position.

Tests of Inner Ear Function

Audiometry (Figure 4.6)

Audiometers vary in complexity but a standard audiogram measures the level of hearing by air and bone conduction. First, using headphones the threshold of hearing is measured at a full range of frequencies from 125 Hz to 8000 Hz. After this the bone conduction is measured using a vibrator placed on the mastoid process. With both tests the non-tested ear will be masked appropriately to prevent sound being heard on that side.

In sensorineural deafness both air and bone conduction will be reduced by the same amount, whereas with a conductive deafness the air conduction will be reduced but the bone conduction will be essentially normal, and this audiogram will show an air-bone gap.

Further audiometry

Impedance audiometry/tympanometry

This is the only type of further audiometry which may be met in general practice or in many hospital audiometry units.

A plug is inserted into the ear canal, sealing it, and

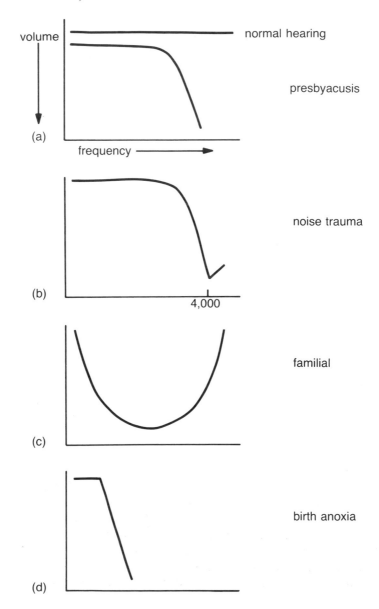

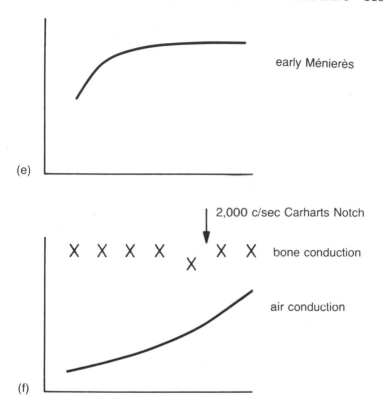

Figure 4.6 Audiometry classical audiograms: (a) to (e), audiograms showing sensorineural hearing loss; (f) conductive deafness in otosclerosis

the pressure in the ear canal can be changed. Sound is transmitted through a channel in the plug and, when the pressure in the meatus is equal to the pressure in the middle ear, the ear drum vibrates maximally and sound will 'enter the middle ear system'. When the pressure is unequal an amount of sound is reflected from the drum proportional to the inequality of pressure. This enables the middle ear pressure to be measured and, in addition, the amount of movement of the middle ear structures can be measured. This will be high in a scarred, thin ear drum and in ossicular discontinuity, and low if the drum is tethered by fluid and in some cases of ossicular fixation.

Speech audiometry, loudness balance, tone decay, and *SISI* are tests used in perceptive/sensorineural deafness. These complex tests are used to distinguish between sensory (inner ear) and neural (VIIIth nerve) deafness to attempt to exclude an acoustic neuroma in cases of unilateral sensorineural deafness.

Vestibular function (Figure 4.7)

Clinical tests

With the eyes shut the body behaves like a paddle steamer, moving forward guided by the equal and opposite action of its balance organs (paddles). When one organ of balance fails the steamer and body will both move towards the affected side, pushed by the unopposed action of the normal 'paddle'.

1 The patient is asked to walk a straight line with the eyes shut, and will veer towards the affected side.

2 When asked to mark time on the spot the patient will rotate towards the affected side.

Nystagmus

The nystagmus caused by disease of the vestibular apparatus has a slow (pathological) component and a

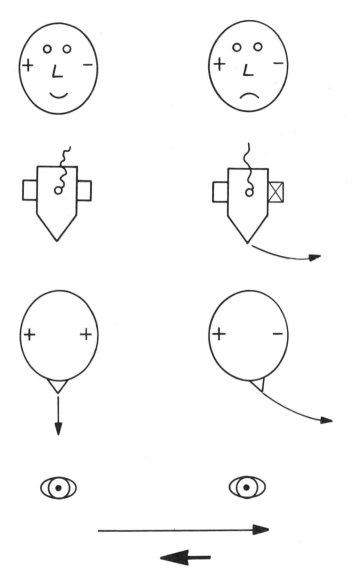

Figure 4.7 Vestibular function – loss of one organ of balance

fast (corrective) component. The eyes are pushed towards the affected side and the fast component is away from it.

By convention the direction of nystagmus is described as that of the fast component.

At first, in the acute phase, nystagmus will be seen with the eye in all positions (third-degree nystagmus). Nystagmus when waning is potentiated by moving the eyes towards the side of the fast component; next the nystagmus will only be visible when the eyes are in the midline and looking towards the side of the fast component (second-degree); and finally, only when the eyes are turned towards the direction of the fast component (first-degree). When clinical nystagmus is absent it may be seen when optic fixation is abolished using Frenzel's glasses or in the dark using an infra-red viewer, or with the eyes shut using an electronystagmograph.

Central nystagmus can be differentiated from peripheral as it may be accentuated by optic fixation.

Electronystagmography

Eye movements can be detected by electrodes enabling nystagmus to be recorded and to be observed in the dark or with the eyes shut. A considerable amount of information can be obtained on the site of disease within the inner ear and central connections of the vestibular system by observing in detail the speed of nystagmus and the conditions under which it is potentiated.

Positional tests

These will be discussed under 'Positional vertigo'. The

patient's head is placed in 'critical positions' and the characteristics of the nystagmus and vertigo, which this induces, indicate whether the disease is of the inner ear or is central.

Caloric tests

It was shown by Ewald, using pigeons, that movement of inner ear fluids in one direction produces movement of the eye in the same direction with a compensatory movement in the opposite direction.

Currents are created in the fluids within the lateral semicircular canals which are made vertical by placing the patient on his back with the head at an angle of 30°. After stimulation with hot and cold water at 44 and 30°C (body temperature ± 7°C), the duration of the nystagmus caused is measured, to show if one vestibular apparatus responds better to stimulation than the other one.

If there is a sensorineural hearing disorder it is almost certain that the disorder of the vestibular apparatus will be on the same side.

Diseases of the Pinna

Absence

It is extremely difficult to construct a new pinna, and a wide variety of surgical techniques have been described. In many cases a plastic prosthetic pinna attached by magnets or glue will provide the best solution to this problem.

Trauma

The pinna may be damaged by bites, when earrings are pulled out, cuts, etc. and will be repaired as appropriate. If a portion of the pinna has been removed and can be found, cleaned and sutured back in place, many will survive.

Blows on the ear may lead to sub-perichondrial bleeding, which if left untreated will either undergo fibrosis, with the development of a cauliflower ear, or will become infected, with dissolution of the cartilage and an even worse deformity. If a haematoma is seen it should be drained, pressure applied with bandages and antibiotics prescribed.

Infection

Spread of infection from a boil in the external meatus or, more commonly, from acute external otitis, may spread to the tissue planes of the pinna with cellulitis followed by the development of a sub-perichondrial abscess which will cause the cartilage to dissolve with a very severe deformity.

If cellulitis develops it must be treated energetically with antibiotics and if an abscess forms it must be drained and the ear bandaged tightly to prevent reaccumulation of the pus and a prolonged course of antibiotics will be given.

Diseases of the External Auditory Meatus

Congenital atresia

One's greatest hope is that this is unilateral rather than bilateral, as surgery to correct any congenital abnormality is extremely difficult and hazardous, both to the inner ear and to the facial nerve. If the disease is unilateral then the patient will be advised against surgery to the abnormal ear.

However, if the disease is bilateral then surgery must be performed, if it can be shown by appropriate X-rays, tomograms and audiometry that there is both a functioning inner ear and also some middle ear spaces which can be reconstructed. The surgery for this is extremely difficult and should, ideally, be carried out only by an otologist who specialises in this form of surgery. This is, beyond all others, an indication to refer patients to a single centre within the country which specialises in this work.

External otitis

This may be part of a generalised skin condition or may be provoked by trauma or the introduction of infected water into the ear.

Symptoms

    1 Itching → pain which may be very severe.

2 Discharge from the ear which may be thin and watery or thick.

3 Slight to moderate deafness. If the ear is cleaned the deafness is slight, and this finding is often of value in distinguishing acute otitis externa from an acute infection of a perforated ear drum when the symptoms will be essentially similar. However the deafness will be more severe, but it may be impossible to clean out the ear adequately to examine the ear drum perfectly.

Treatment

1 Cleaning of the ear – by dry mopping in the surgery or suction in an ENT clinic.

2 Swab for bacterial and fungal culture and sensitivities.

3 Appropriate antibiotic/steroid ear drops plus an antifungal if indicated.

4 It is rarely necessary to administer systemic antibiotics unless there is swelling of the pinna suggesting the development of perichondritis. As mentioned above, this must be treated aggressively and, if an abscess forms, it must be drained and a bandage applied to the ear to prevent a reaccumulation of pus. Antibiotics must be given in these cases.

Furuncle (boil)

A boil forms in a hair follicle in the outer part of the meatus and is extremely painful as the skin has no room to stretch in this site. Treatment is with antibiotics and pain may be relieved by the insertion of an ichthammol and glycerine wick, which is hygroscopic and absorbs water from the boil, reducing the pressure within it. Occasionally it may be necessary to drain the abscess.

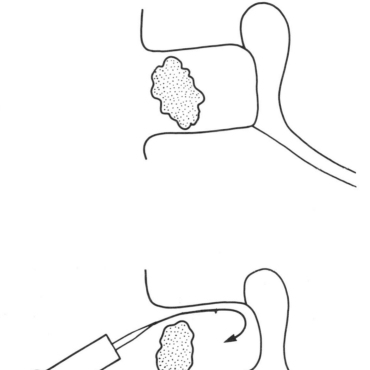

Figure 4.8 Ear syringing

Wax

This is almost certainly the commonest cause of a moderate conductive deafness. Diagnosis is easy and syringing curative (Figure 4.8). Wax is an antiseptic, and the skin of the ear canal migrates peripherally carrying wax out of the external auditory meatus. Self-cleaning of wax, using cotton buds etc., tends to push wax back into the ear canal and should be discouraged.

The technique of syringing is important. A wide variety of ear syringes may be used with tap water which must be at body temperature to prevent vertigo from caloric effects. The jet of water must be aimed at a wall of the meatus, never at the wax, or the wax may be blasted through the ear drum. Most often the wax will have settled to the floor of the meatus leaving a gap between the wax and canal wall superiorly, and the water will be aimed at the roof of the meatus. It will then pass behind the wax and force it out of the canal. After this the ear is mopped and dried.

On occasions proprietary wax softeners or olive oil may be used before syringing to soften hard and impacted wax.

Diseases of the Ear Drum

Viral myringitis

During an upper respiratory tract infection the patient develops severe earache with some deafness followed by a scanty bloody discharge. On examination there will be evidence of blood blisters on the ear drum and on the canal wall, and there may be an effusion into the middle ear with a conductive hearing loss.

Treatment

Analgesics will be necessary, and antibiotics should be given to prevent secondary infection. Nasal decongestant therapy will allow an effusion to drain via the eustachian tube.

Unequal pressure on the two sides of the ear drum

This occurs when there is an obstruction of the eustachian tube with absorption of air from the middle ear space and development of a negative pressure. This causes the ear drum to be sucked in, and its normal vibrations are reduced with a significant conductive hearing loss. In children this negative pressure develops when adenoids obstruct the eustachian tube, and in adults a diagnosis of carcinoma of the nasopharynx must be made until proved otherwise.

On occasions this pressure change may be acute, as when descending in an aeroplane with the eustachian tubes blocked by an upper respiratory tract infection. The increasing atmospheric pressure results in a severe pushing in of the ear drums with pain and a serous effusion, with, on occasions, bleeding into the middle ear.

Divers experience the reverse effect on surfacing, with a blowing-out of the ear drums with blood in the middle ear and occasionally rupture of the ear drum.

Traumatic rupture

A blow on the side of the head may rupture the ear drum and perforations may be extremely large. However, even large perforations will heal if the ear does not become infected, and the patients should be advised to keep the ear dry and to report to the hospital if there is any evidence of discharge. Some advocate the prescription of antibiotics for all these patients to prevent ear infection which may result in the perforation becoming permanent and the development of the safe form of chronic suppurative otitis media.

Chronic suppurative otitis media

There are two forms of this disease: first, safe and second, unsafe (see Table 4.1); both are characterised by:

1 Deafness.

2 Discharge.

3 Defect in the tympanic membrane.

Safe chronic suppurative otitis media

This develops in a patient who has a perforated ear drum, either from pus in acute otitis media bursting outwards or trauma bursting inwards. If in acute otitis media the discharge of pus dries up quickly and, if a traumatic perforation does not become infected, then the perforations will heal rapidly with a restoration of normal ear drum function. However, if discharge persists, in acute otitis media, or if a traumatic

Table 4.1 *Comparison of two forms of chronic suppurative otitis media*

	Safe	Unsafe
Discharge	Thin Intermittent Copious Inoffensive	Thick Continuous Scanty Offensive
Deafness	Conductive	Conductive – may be sensorineural
Defect	Pars tensa Central	Pars flaccida Marginal
Complications	Nil	Death, brain abscess, meningitis, extradural abscess, vertigo and inner ear damage, facial nerve paralysis
Surgery	The patient may choose: Myringoplasty Tympanoplasty (drum and ossicles)	Surgery must be carried out: Mastoidectomy

perforation becomes infected, the discharge of pus through the perforation prevents normal healing, but the ear drum heals abnormally with the skin on the outside healing with the mucosa on the inside around the fibrous drum of the pars tensa. Once this has

happened the perforation has been 'sealed' and there
will be no further tendency for it to heal (Figure 4.9).

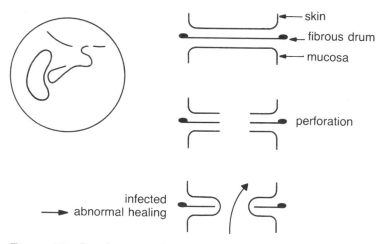

*Figure 4.9   Development of a permanent central perforation in safe
chronic suppurative otitis media*

Characteristics

1 *Deafness* – this is conductive and the amount of
   hearing loss depends on the size of the perforation and whether the ossicular chain has been
   damaged.

2 *Discharge* – (a) intermittent, occurs when the
   patient gets the ear wet or gets a cold; (b)
   copious; (c) thin, mucoid; (d) non-offensive.

3 *Defect* – the perforation is of the pars tensa and
   is central, which means that there is a rim of
   ear drum all around it. The infection in acute
   otitis media is contained behind the pars tensa
   by folds of mucosa around the ossicular chain
   which prevent infection from spreading to the

attic and thence to the mastoid air cell system. Acute otitis media always ruptures through the pars tensa, as does a traumatic perforation. The size of the perforation varies from relatively small to sub-total, in which almost all the pars tensa has been lost apart from the rim of drum and some drum around the handle of the malleus.

Treatment

The intermittent discharge can be dried up by appropriate antibiotic/steroid ear drops, and only rarely will systemic antibiotics be needed. An audiogram will then be performed.

The patient should then be told what can be offered by surgery, and what will happen if surgery is not performed. If surgery is not performed the patient will continue to be deaf on the affected side and have intermittent discharge, which can be dried up rapidly by drops. The patient should be told that there is no risk to life or to health, and that there should be no significant progression of the deafness. The patient must then be told that if surgery is performed to repair the ear drum, there is an 80–90 per cent chance of success with an improvement in the hearing and a cessation of the attacks of discharge. All the patients who are to have ear surgery must be warned that there is a slight but significant chance of increasing the hearing loss, and that in a very small number of cases inner ear damage may occur with a 'dead ear'.

In safe chronic otitis media the patient can and must be allowed to decide if he feels that his symptoms justify surgery. Often patients prefer the relatively mild symptoms of deafness and occasional episodes of discharge to surgery once they have been assured that there are no serious sequelae to the disease.

Surgery

Myringoplasty – repair of the ear drum

Fascia from the temporalis muscle is used to repair the defect and numerous techniques have been described for the operation. The graft may be placed on the inner surface of the ear drum supported by absorbable gelatine sponge in the middle ear or on the outside between the fibrous drum and the skin. All techniques should offer an 80–90 per cent chance of closing the perforation.

Tympanoplasty – repair of the drum and ossicular chain

The reconstruction will be determined by the defect in the ossicular chain which is found at operation. The long process of the incus, which articulates with the stapes, is most often damaged by disease as its blood supply is poor and pressure of pus on the vessels may result in avascular necrosis. If a significant proportion of the body of the incus remains, it can be removed and fashioned into a prosthesis to lie between the handle of malleus and the stapes. Homograft ossicles, plastic and wire prostheses and reinforced cartilage struts have also been used and, in very gross defects of the ear drum and ossicular chain, homograft drums with ossicles attached may be used.

Unsafe chronic suppurative otitis media

This condition is life-threatening and is associated with the development of a cholesteatoma. The underlying pathology is chronic negative pressure in the middle ear from eustachian tube obstruction.

The pars flaccida in the upper part of the ear drum is composed of two layers – skin and mucous membrane –

unlike the pars tensa which has skin and mucous membrane separated by the fibrous drum. The pars flaccida is therefore more susceptible to negative pressure, and becomes sucked in and retracted to form an attic dimple.

The skin of the ear drum and ear canal migrates peripherally all the time and, like all skin, sheds keratin from its superficial layer. The sheet of migrating keratin moves superiorly and becomes trapped within the attic dimple which is also lined by desquamating skin and fills up with dead keratin. By 'onion-skin' accumulation of keratin the sucked-in invaginated pars flaccida becomes a much larger pocket or sac and this sac extends progressively into the middle ear air spaces; this is a cholesteatoma (Figure 4.10).

The feature of a cholesteatoma which makes it so dangerous is that the outer surface of the sac can erode any bone with which it comes into contact, and it can invade the cranial cavity, inner ear and facial nerve.

Many patients will not present until complications have developed and these include intra-cranial spread, facial nerve paralysis or vertigo and sensorineural deafness. This form of chronic suppurative otitis media is normally painless and the development of pain indicates that the dura has been exposed.

Characteristics

1 *Discharge* (a) continuous – the discharge is present all the time and there are no prolonged periods of freedom from it; (b) thick – moist infected keratin oozes from the neck of the cholesteatoma sac; (c) scanty; (d) offensive.

2 *Deafness* – conductive, the degree of hearing loss depends on the amount of destruction of

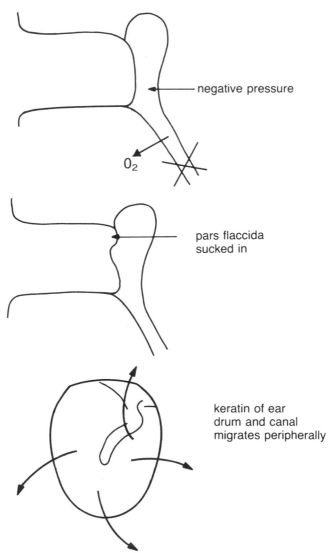

Figure 4.10   Development of a cholesteatoma in unsafe chronic suppurative otitis media (a)

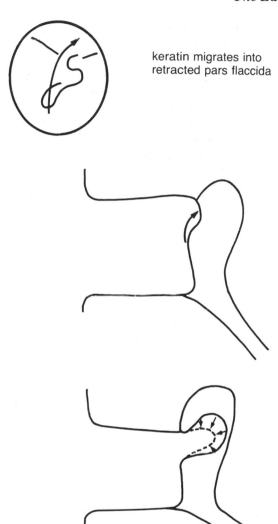

keratin migrates into
retracted pars flaccida

*Figure 4.10 Development of a cholesteatoma in unsafe chronic
suppurative otitis media (b)*

middle ear structures. If the cholesteatoma has invaded the inner ear, then the deafness may be sensorineural with vertigo.

3 *Defect* – this is of the pars flaccida and, although it looks like a perforation, it is in reality the neck of the keratin-filled cholesteatoma sac which extends into the middle ear and mastoid air spaces. The defect is marginal and there is no rim of ear drum around it.

Investigation

1 An X-ray will be performed to show if there has been any significant bone erosion by the cholesteatoma.

2 Many surgeons perform suction clearance under anaesthetic. At operation suction is used to remove the keratin from the cholesteatoma sac and, if the sac is shallow complete clearance may be achieved. In this way the patient's ear may be kept clean. This technique may occasionally be used for treatment in elderly patients not suitable for more extensive surgery.

Treatment

Patients must be warned that they have a life-threatening disease and that surgery must be performed.

Obviously if a patient presents with a complication then surgery will be carried out immediately.

The operation of mastoidectomy will be performed and a variety of techniques have been described. The air cell system of the middle ear and mastoid process cannot be reached for removal of the cholesteatoma until its bony covering has been removed; this removal constitutes a mastoidectomy. In a majority of cases, having exenterated the mastoid air cells the bony wall between the ear canal and the mastoid air spaces will be removed so that a large cavity is created which can be reached via the external auditory meatus for cleaning and the prevention of reaccumulation of keratin debris. Once a patient has had a radical mastoidectomy of this type he must be seen once or twice each year for cleaning of the cavity which has lost its 'self-cleaning mechanism'.

It is now possible, on occasions, to reconstruct ears which have been severely damaged by chronic ear infection, but the absolute rule is that all middle ear infection and cholesteatoma must be cleared before reconstruction can be contemplated.

Scarring

The ear drums may be thickened with calcified plaques following repeated middle ear infections. This can interfere with ear drum vibrations and cause some slight deafness. Scarring may also cause thin atrophic areas of the ear drum which can balloon out like a spinnaker when the middle ear pressure changes. These segments, too, may result in some conductive hearing loss.

Abnormalities of the Middle Ear

Fluid in the middle ear

The accumulation of all forms of fluid in the middle ear

is considered in detail in the section on the adenoids.

1 Pus – in acute otitis media.

2 Thin fluid – in serous otitis media from eustachian tube obstruction. If this occurs in an adult, then a diagnosis of carcinoma of the nasopharynx must be made until proved otherwise.

3 Thick fluid (glue) – in obstruction of the eustachian tube with occasional episodes of infection.

Blood

A haemotympanum may occur after trauma in which the middle ear is filled with blood, causing a significant conductive deafness. In cases of trauma it must be determined by audiometry if the deafness is from a haemotympanum alone or from a combination of haemotympanum and inner ear damage.

Antibiotics may be given to prevent infection of the blood, and nasal decongestants may aid the drainage of the blood via the eustachian tube.

Adhesions

These may form after repeated middle ear infection and can tether the ossicular chain which can be freed at surgery. On occasions very thin sheets of Teflon may be inserted to prevent re-formation of the adhesions.

Polypi

An aural polyp is a swollen mass of middle ear mucous

membrane which will protrude through a perforation. Aural polypi can be removed surgically but extreme care must be exercised in their removal to avoid damage to the middle ear structures. After removal the perforation will be treated on merit.

On very rare occasions a 'polyp' may be a glomus jugulare tumour of chemodectoma tissue arising from the medial wall of the middle ear, and removal of these may be accompanied by severe haemorrhage.

Disorders of the Ossicles

Dislocation

Dislocation occurs after a head injury and commonly the incus separates from the stapes. This causes a significant conductive deafness and on tympanometry a hyper-mobile ear drum and ossicular chain will be found. Treatment is by surgery, in which the middle ear is opened and a bone chip placed between the incus and stapes to reconstitute the ossicular chain.

Avascular necrosis

During an acute middle ear infection the pressure of the pus occludes the fine vessels which supply the ossicular chain causing avascular necrosis. The most susceptible part of the chain is the long process of the incus which articulates with the stapes.

The patient, who will also, on most occasions, have a perforated ear drum, will suffer significant conductive hearing loss worse than a patient who has a perforation alone. Treatment will be by the operation of tympanoplasty to repair the ear drum and to reconstruct the ossicular chain by reshaping the body of the incus to fit between the malleus and the stapes.

Otosclerosis

This is a familial condition causing conductive hearing loss which is often bilateral, although one ear may present before the other. The disease tends to occur more frequently in women, and the first evidence of deafness may present during pregnancy.

Pathology

In front of the oval window, which contains the stapes, is a fissure in the otic capsule, named the fissure ante fenestram (fissure in front of the window). Something, as yet unknown, causes a growth of bone from this fissure and eventually it encroaches from the edge of the oval window onto the stapes, fixing it and causing a progressive conductive hearing loss. (Figure 4.11)

Symptoms

> 1 Progressive conductive hearing loss, which may be asymmetrical.
>
> 2 Paracusis – the ability to hear sounds better in a noisy environment. This is because the patient is not able to hear the background noise but can hear the voices raised above it.

Signs

A normal ear drum but, on occasions, a slight pink

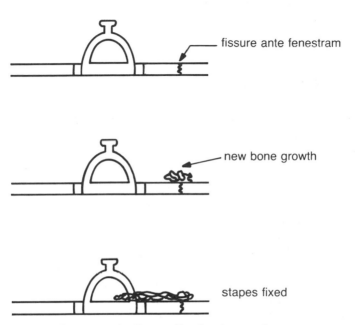

stapes in oval window

fissure ante fenestram

new bone growth

stapes fixed

Figure 4.11 Stapes fixation in otosclerosis

flushing of the posterior superior quadrant of the pars tensa may be seen – the flamingo flush – from the hyperaemic otosclerotic bone glowing through the ear drum.

Treatment

The patient must be advised that two treatments are possible: first, a hearing aid which will improve the hearing significantly; second, the operation of stapedectomy in which, after the middle ear has been opened, the stapes is removed and replaced with a plastic or metal strut to reconstruct the ossicular chain.

The patient should be told that, although the chance of
restoration of the hearing by stapedectomy is more
than 90 per cent, there is a 1–2 per cent chance of inner
ear damage with severe perceptive hearing loss, which
may amount to a 'dead ear'.

Patients must be told clearly of the two alternatives
and allowed to choose between them, but many
patients dislike hearing aids intensely and, despite the
slight but definite risk, will choose surgery.

Inner Ear Diseases

The intimate relationship within the inner ear of the
cochlea – the organ of hearing – and the vestibular
apparatus – the organ of balance – means that any
disease within the inner ear can cause both deafness
and vertigo. Either one of the two symptoms can occur
in isolation, but some disorders may produce both
deafness and vertigo, although one symptom may
predominate.

Perceptive–sensorineural deafness

(Sensory = inner ear deafness; neural = VIIIth nerve
deafness)

This deafness may be of sudden onset or gradually
progressive, and it may be unilateral or bilateral.
Speech intelligibility is reduced more in high-frequency
deafness than in the less common low-frequency
hearing loss, as the loss of the high-frequency consonants is of much great significance than that of the
low-frequency vowels.

Most disorders which cause sensorineural hearing loss are untreatable, and help for the patient is by the provision of a hearing aid, lip-reading classes, education and rehabilitation. Medical and surgical treatments can arrest the progress and occasionally reverse the hearing loss of Menière's disease. Acute sensorineural hearing loss, caused by either a vascular accident or a virus infection, represents an acute otological emergency and unless treatment with vasodilators and/or steroids is given immediately it will be of no value. If, during strenuous exercise, the round window membrane between the inner ear and middle ear ruptures, then urgent surgical treatment is required to arrest and reverse the progress of the hearing loss and vertigo.

Cochlear implants are under development, but at present they are only of value in providing some auditory signals to those with complete bilateral deafness. One must be optimistic about their future, but much more research and development is necessary before they are widely available and of benefit to other groups of hearing-impaired patients.

Vertigo

Many patients present with symptoms such as giddy turns, dizziness or attacks of loss of balance, and from this rag-bag of symptoms one must identify the patient with true vertigo. In true vertigo the patient has a hallucination of movement, either of the patient within the environment or of the environment around the patient and, although classically this is rotatory, it may be from side to side or backwards and forwards.

Eighty-five per cent of cases of true vertigo are

caused by peripheral disease of the inner ear or VIIIth nerve, and only 15 per cent are central with disease inside the cranial cavity. Central causes will not be discussed here at length, except to state that if vertigo is accompanied by eye symptoms and headache it may be part of the migraine complex, and if a patient becomes unconscious after an acute attack of vertigo it could be due to temporal lobe epilepsy. In most other cases of central vertigo there will be evidence of other neurological symptoms and signs.

When deprived of function of one organ of balance, as mentioned above, the patient will behave like a paddle steamer deprived of one paddle and will veer towards the affected side. This forms the basis of a number of clinical tests. Patients will usually compensate for the loss of one balance organ after 6–8 weeks, or longer in older patients. However, a patient cannot compensate for the constant input of abnormal information from a severely damaged vestibular apparatus. This explains the rationale behind the performance of the operation of labyrinthectomy in patients with intractable vertigo, when one balance organ has been severely damaged but not completely destroyed, to remove the last remnants of labyrinthine function to allow the patient to compensate.

Deafness alone

Deafness in children

This form of deafness is almost invariably incurable. It may be familial, acquired in pregnancy or in the perinatal period, or it may develop in childhood. Although the deafness cannot be cured the quality of life of the patient depends on the deafness being recognised as early as possible, so that all the necessary help can be given in the form of hearing aids and appropriate education. A hearing aid can be fitted to a child at the age of 6 months.

Causes

Familial

Numerous syndromes which include deafness have been described, and the nature of the deafness is often well known by the family and readily diagnosed. Genetic counselling must be made available for the parents.

During pregnancy

1 *Drugs*. Care must be taken in the prescription of drugs to pregnant women as a large number have been blamed for fetal abnormalities.

2 *Infection*
   (a) *Rubella – German measles*. It is vitally important to vaccinate all girls who have not had German measles, to avoid this preventable cause of fetal abnormalities. If a women develops rubella during pregnancy an abortion will often be suggested. However, the infection may be subclinical and only detected by a high titre of antibodies. This will show that rubella has caused the abnormalities, and indicates that other children in the future will not be affected.
   (b) *Syphillis*. This should be picked up on routine serology.

3　*Toxaemia*

4　*Antepartum　haemorrhage* ⎫ These problems with the pregnancy may give rise to fetal abnormalities which can include deafness.

Perinatal

At birth fetal trauma and prolonged periods of anoxia may severely damage the inner ears. Within the immediate postnatal period, neonatal jaundice may be responsible for profound bilateral hearing loss.

In childhood

1　*Meningitis* – cerebrospinal fluid is continuous with the perilymph of the inner ear via the cochlear aqueduct; therefore meningitis can spread to the inner ear causing a suppurative labyrinthitis with severe or total sensorineural hearing loss, which is often bilateral. Early diagnosis and treatment of meningitis is essential to prevent this terrible complication.

2　*Infectious fevers* – The viruses of mumps, measles and influenza may all damage the inner ear causing a sudden onset of severe sensorineural hearing loss. This is rarely, if ever, diagnosed in the acute phase but on rare occasions, if vasodilator therapy is given, some improvement in the hearing loss may be obtained. It is usually diagnosed relatively late and is therefore untreatable but, happily, deafness caused by these infections is almost always unilateral.

3 *Trauma* – trauma to the head, particularly when it is severe enough to cause a fracture through the temporal bone, may result in a severe or total hearing loss which is almost always unilateral on the side of the injury.

Diagnosis

It is vitally important that all children, and in particular those who are at risk, are screened most carefully by competent workers to diagnose deafness as early as possible.

'At-risk registers' were available, and included all children who had a family history of deafness and abnormalities in pregnancy or in the neonatal period. These children were obviously screened even more intensively than other children, but these at-risk registers are not now widely available.

If any doubt exists as to the level of hearing, then objective hearing tests are available to determine the true level of hearing without the need for patient co-operation. These include an acoustic cradle which can be used to monitor the neonate's reaction to sound; a computerised audiometer which measures the post-auricular muscle response when a child is exposed to sound; and electrocochleography when, under an anaesthetic, an electrode is passed through the ear drum onto the bone overlying the cochlea to measure its response, and that of the VIIIth nerve, to sound.

Management

A detailed description of the management of a severely deaf child is beyond the scope of this book, and only a brief outline will be given. Children must be under the care of a deaf children's clinic and after the true level of hearing loss has been determined, appropriate hearing aids will be provided. Continuing advice will also be given on the education of the child: whether he should attend a normal school, a normal school with a department for deaf children, or perhaps a special deaf children's school. Appropriate psychological and psychiatric guidance must also be available for both patient and parents. Peripatetic teachers of the deaf will arrange to visit the family in the home, and will advise on all problems relating to the deafness. Support for the whole family must be provided by the general practitioner.

Noise-induced hearing loss

It is now well known that high-intensity sound can damage the hearing, and noise-induced hearing loss is a recognised and compensatable industrial injury. At first, the damage is at the higher frequencies, and 4000 Hz is the first to be affected. However, if exposure to noise continues, the lower frequencies will eventually be affected and the patient will experience increasing problems with speech discrimination. All workers in noisy employment must be fully advised on the dangers of exposure to noise and must be provided with appropriate ear protection. However, it is sad to say that many workers so advised will still decline to wear ear protection. There is no cure for this form of deafness and, although a hearing aid may be of some limited benefit, the loss of consonants associated with high-frequency hearing loss means that speech intelligibility suffers considerably.

Presbyacusis – deafness in old age

Presbyacusis (old man's hearing) is the deafness which develops in old age as a result of exposure to noise, and inner ear degeneration. Hearing loss is for the high frequencies which severely affect speech intelligibility as described above; old patients in addition may have some central problems with the interpretation of perceived sounds.

The patients suffer a number of problems, including in many cases a lack of understanding and sympathy from relatives and friends, who often force patients to obtain hearing aids which may be of limited value.

A very large number of old patients will refuse to wear a body-worn hearing aid which offers a better quality of sound amplification, and they will insist on the provision of a small, behind-the-ear hearing aid. Some very high-quality behind-the-ear aids are available in the private sector, but at a cost of many hundreds of pounds, and the aids provided by the health service, although of acceptable quality, would retail at a much lower price and the quality of sound amplification is far from perfect. In addition these aids are difficult to adjust if the patient has arthritic fingers or anything less than perfect manual dexterity.

Patients assume that the moment the hearing aid is inserted the hearing will return as if by magic, and are invariably disappointed by the quality of amplification. Patient education is of the greatest importance and is not always provided; as a result, many hearing aids remain unworn.

The aim must be to provide patients with high-quality hearing aids and enough information to ensure that the patient obtains optimum benefit from the aid. However, no elderly patient with presbyacusis will regain normal hearing by using a hearing aid, and both family and friends must be educated and told that it is essential to talk to the deaf person face to face so that lip-reading can be employed and to articulate clearly in a firm, but not loud, voice.

Patients with presbyacusis need care, sympathy and understanding which, even in the best of families, is difficult to provide.

Deafness and vertigo

Trauma

Direct trauma

Direct trauma to the skull will result in a spectrum of damage to the inner ear from a reversible concussion to a total loss of inner ear function, associated with a fracture through the temporal bone. Diagnosis will not be difficult.

Treatment

The vertigo can be controlled in the acute phase with labyrinthine sedatives, and the administration of vasodilators may help to minimise damage and hasten recovery. In cases of intractable vertigo from severe damage to the vestibular apparatus, a labyrinthectomy may be performed to destroy the remnants of labyrinthine function and to remove the constant input of abnormal information from the diseased organ of balance, to allow the patient to compensate.

Round window membrane rupture

The history in this condition is almost diagnostic. A patient complains of a sudden onset of hearing loss with vertigo when undertaking some heavy, physical exercise.

During this exercise there is a rise in intracranial pressure and, as the CSF is continuous with the perilymph of the inner ear via the cochlear aqueduct, this rise in pressure is transmitted to the inner ear which bursts through the delicate round window membrane which lies between the inner ear and the middle ear. The hearing loss and vertigo may fluctuate with a progressive deterioration.

Treatment

When the diagnosis of round window membrane rupture is suspected the patient should be given labyrinthine sedatives to control the vertigo and should be referred immediately to hospital where the middle ear will be opened and the ruptured round window membrane patched with fat. This should control the vertigo and prevent further deterioration in the hearing, which may, on occasions, show some recovery.

Vascular

Sudden occlusion of the internal auditory artery which often occurs in an older patient will cause acute sensorineural hearing loss. The deafness may on occasions be accompanied by vertigo, but this is not common. It has been said that this type of sudden deafness represents a warning of a more serious vascular accident to come, either coronary or cerebrovascular.

Treatment

If this is to be of any value it must be given early, but even so the results are uncertain. When seen within 24 hours the patient will be treated by aggressive vasodilatation, which may include a histamine drip, the inhalation of carbon dioxide or a stellate ganglion block. In addition the patient will be given oral vasodilators and steroids on a reducing dose for 2–3 weeks.

Patients with sudden sensorineural hearing loss represent an acute otological emergency and must be referred to hospital immediately for treatment, even though this treatment may not always be successful.

Infection

Bacterial

Meningitis

Cerebrospinal fluid is continuous with the perilymph of the inner ear via the cochlear aqueduct, and the infection of meningitis can spread along this route to cause a suppurative labyrinthitis. The deafness may be total and bilateral and, once it has occurred, there is no cure. It is therefore essential to diagnose and treat meningitis urgently, to prevent this appalling complication.

Chronic suppurative otitis media

Unsafe chronic otitis media with cholesteatoma is described elsewhere. The cholesteatoma sac can erode the bony wall between the middle ear and inner ear, usually into the lateral semicircular canal giving rise to vertigo and progressive sensorineural hearing loss. An important physical sign of this erosion of the inner ear is the 'fistula test'. A finger is pressed onto the tragus of the ear and this pressure is transmitted via the external auditory meatus through the cholesteatoma sac to the inner ear, causing movement of the inner ear fluids and momentary vertigo with nystagmus. If this test is positive in a case of unsafe chronic suppurative otitis media, one must assume that there is a fistula into the inner ear and urgent referral to hospital is vital. When diagnosed a mastoidectomy will be performed immediately, but management of the fistula into the lateral semicircular canal is still the subject of heated and complex otological debate.

Viral

A complication of mumps, measles and influenza is a viral labyrinthitis with a severe and often total hearing loss which is, happily, almost always unilateral. Transient vertigo may occur at the onset of the deafness during the acute illness, but is not always noticed as the child may not complain of vertigo but only of the nausea and vomiting which accompany it.

Herpes zoster can affect the ear, giving rise to the Ramsay Hunt syndrome which comprises sensorineural hearing loss with vertigo, facial nerve paralysis and pain in the ear with vesicles in the meatus or on the palate. The deafness may be severe and can, on occasions, be helped by vasodilators; the facial nerve paralysis may be complete. It is thought to be dangerous to give steroids in these cases as they may allow the virus to spread to adjacent cranial nerves.

Spirochaetal

Syphilis is, perhaps, not quite as rare as it was, and if the patient suffers from persistent vertigo with a progressive, bilateral sensory neural hearing loss, then serology must always be done to exclude syphilitic labyrinthitis.

Drugs

Ototoxic drugs are now well known and include the amino glycoside antibiotics. Gentamicin is the only one of these which is now administered regularly systemically and, as it is cleared by the kidneys, it should not be given to patients with renal failure. In addition, the very old and the very young do not clear the drug normally and, as with all patients, it should be administered only when blood levels can be monitored. If facilities are not available to measure the blood levels of gentamicin then the serum creatinine should be measured as this has a linear relationship with the blood levels of the drug.

Other ototoxic drugs include aspirin and, if administered to a patient, the doctor will recognise the onset of tinnitus and a little sensory hearing loss as a warning of overdosage. However, self-medication poses perhaps a greater threat to the inner ear, as many patients taking a proprietary medicine containing large amounts of aspirin will not relate the tinnitus and progressive hearing loss to the medicine.

Ménière's disease

This disease presents most commonly before the age of 50, and the attacks of vertigo are associated with emotional or physical stress. The patient suffers from severe spontaneous attacks of rotatory vertigo which come on without warning and are accompanied by nausea and vomiting. Each attack lasts for minutes or hours and the attacks often occur in clusters, which last days or weeks separated by periods free from vertigo lasting months or even years.

The patient suffers a progressive sensorineural hearing loss which is at first for the low frequencies but eventually involves the whole frequency range, and tinnitus which may be extremely disturbing. The tinnitus and hearing loss both deteriorate during attacks of vertigo, and although the level of hearing may improve after the attacks it never regains fully its 'pre-attack level'.

Patients also complain of a sensation of fulness in the affected ear and diplacusis – the hearing of sounds at an abnormal pitch on the affected side. The disease is unilateral in 85 per cent of cases, and the disorder is due to an excess of endolymph within the membranous inner ear.

This abnormality is thought to be caused by a vasoconstriction in the stria vascularis of the cochlea in which endolymph is certainly produced and possibly absorbed.

Diagnosis

This is made on the history of the pattern of the attacks of vertigo with the accompanying symptoms and the finding of a hearing loss on audiogram and labyrinthine dysfunction on caloric tests.

It is said that classical Ménière's disease is uncommon, and this is probably true, but a large number of 'Ménière's-like diseases' exist, which are essentially similar to the classical Ménière's disease and respond identically to treatment but vary in some detail from the classical description.

Treatment

First the patients must be reassured, as they are convinced that they have some serious intracranial problem such as a vascular accident or tumour. Second, many specialists utilise a low-salt, low-fluid diet and a number of vitamin preparations. It is certainly wise to advise the patient to cut down and, if possible, to stop smoking, as this causes vasoconstriction and may exacerbate the disease, but if the patient is seriously disturbed by giving up smoking a compromise must be reached.

Labyrinthine sedatives may be of help in controlling the attacks of vertigo but they tend to have unpleasant side-effects and patients are often not happy to take these for prolonged periods.

Betahistine causes a local vasodilatation within the inner ear and appears to be specific for Ménière's and Ménière's-like diseases. A high dose may have to be given at first and then this is titrated to a minimum maintenance dose which may have to be continued for months or even years.

It has been estimated that approximately 90 per cent of patients can be controlled by reassurance and drugs, but on occasions surgery will be necessary to control intractable vertigo. In the vast majority of those who require surgery the hearing will be essentially useless, and a labyrinthectomy will be performed. However, a small number of patients with intractable vertigo have useful hearing and a number of sophisticated surgical procedures are available to control the vertigo and to preserve the hearing. These include drainage of the endolymphatic sac via a mastoidectomy approach and sectioning the vestibular part of the VIIIth nerve.

Acoustic neuroma

Any patient with unilateral, sensorineural hearing loss with balance probems must be diagnosed as having an acoustic neuroma until proved otherwise. All such patients must be fully investigated to make a diagnosis and to exclude this tumour which, if it is to be removed without significant morbidity, must be removed when it is small.

An acoustic neuroma should present classically with a slowly progressive sensorineural hearing loss with a generalised unsteadiness, rather than episodic vertigo, but atypical presentations are common and all cases must be fully investigated. However, in the elderly the morbidity of surgery for an acoustic neuroma is considerable, and many believe that unilateral, sensorineural hearing loss with balance problems should not be investigated in the old as the morbidity of surgery might be greater than that of the untreated tumour. It should, of course, go without saying that each case must be treated on merit.

Vertigo alone

Spontaneous — vestibular neuronitis

This condition, thought to be due to a virus, may occasionally sweep through a school or other establishment, and has been known as acute epidemic vertigo. An otherwise healthy patient experiences a sudden onset of severe rotatory vertigo with nausea and vomiting and will exhibit nystagmus in the acute illness. The symptoms will gradually settle over a period of several weeks, although very rarely there may be a recurrence.

Treatment

In the acute phase, treatment with labyrinthine sedatives is essential and these may have to be given intramuscularly if vomiting is severe.

Positional

Benign positional vertigo

In this condition the patient experiences vertigo when the head is in a critical position, usually when lying flat with the head turned to one side. The diagnosis can be made by performing the positional test. Here, the patient's head is put into the critical position. After a latent period, he will exhibit nystagmus with vertigo, but the nystagmus is of short duration. This test is fatiguable in that it cannot be performed again without pausing for several minutes.

This pattern of nystagmus differentiates it from a central positional vertigo. Here, when the head is put in the critical position, nystagmus occurs immediately and is continuous for as long as the head is in the critical position. This test is not fatiguable.

Treatment

The patient should be told the nature of the disorder, which is thought to be due to a minor lesion of one of the static organs of balance. Patients tend to learn a way of lying down without provoking the vertigo, and labyrinthine sedatives may be of help for the patient to take when he goes to bed. The condition is usually prolonged but tends to be self-limiting.

Vertebrobasilar insufficiency

Classically, this occurs in the patient with either cervical, spine or arterial disease who looks up at a high object, kinking the neck and with it the vertebral arteries, which travel up the vertebrarterial canals in the cervical vertebrae. This momentarily cuts off the circulation to the inner ears causing temporary labyrinthine dysfunction with vertigo. However, it is more commonly seen in older patients who suddenly rise from lying or sitting and experience momentary cardiac inefficiency with a similar loss of blood supply to the vestibular apparatus. These patients should be told the nature of the problem and advised to get out of bed in a series of separate movements, rather than one overall movement.

First, sit up in bed, then sit on the edge of the bed before standing up. Then move off.

If the patient understands the nature of the problem he can learn to live with it.

Conclusions

The most important aid to the diagnosis of vertigo is the history – the pattern and duration of the attacks, provoking features and associated symptoms, etc. Although a general practitioner should make a provisional diagnosis and begin treatment, all cases of persistent vertigo, with or without deafness, should be investigated at some time in a Department of Otoneurology to confirm the diagnosis and to exclude an acoustic neuroma.

Tinnitus

Tinnitus causes patients great distress and it remains untreatable in almost all cases. Two forms exist: the rare objective tinnitus, in which the noise can also be heard by the doctor, and the very much more common subjective tinnitus, in which the patient alone can hear the noise, which may be very loud, unilateral or bilateral and described as the noise of machinery, hissing, whistling, etc.

Objective tinnitus

Palatal myoclonus

This is almost always psychosomatic but rarely can be caused by a lesion in the brainstem. The palate moves up and down at a rate of 120–140 beats per minute, causing the eustachian tube to open and close, and this is heard as a clicking sound.

Vascular

Patients with a conductive deafness can often 'hear their own pulse' in an ear isolated from outside noise. However, severe pulsatile tinnitus may be caused by a vascular malformation, aberrant vessel or vascular tumour. In severe cases arteriography may be indicated, and an abnormal vessel or glomus jugulare tumour will be treated on merit.

Subjective tinnitus

Tinnitus is a relatively non-specific symptom of ear damage. In some cases of Menière's disease, medical or surgical treatment may improve the symptom but tinnitus from all other causes is essentially untreatable.

The patient should not be filled with useless drugs and false hopes, but should be told of the nature of the symptom and that, although no specific treatment is available, there is a tendency for the nuisance of tinnitus to decrease as the patient gets used to it. The patient must be told to avoid further damage to the ear from noise, etc., as this will tend to worsen the tinnitus.

In attempts to find a cure for tinnitus, a wide range of drugs given orally and intravenously have been tried, but none has given consistently good results. The treatment of tinnitus therefore remains one of the major unsolved problems in ENT.

Patients who find difficulty in getting to sleep may be helped by a clock radio which turns itself off after the patient has fallen asleep listening to soft music. There is also an increasing interest in tinnitus maskers, which are worn like a hearing aid and make a less unpleasant sound than the tinnitus. However, tinnitus remains a severe and unsolved problem causing great distress to many patients.

CHAPTER 5

FACIAL NERVE PARALYSIS

Paralysis of one side of the face is an extremely unpleasant cosmetic deformity and bilateral facial nerve paralysis is quite grotesque. The defect is almost entirely cosmetic, although there is some risk of damage to the cornea if the eye lids cannot close completely to protect it.

Causes

Trauma

Fracture of the temporal bone

Facial nerve paralysis may be immediate or delayed. If delayed it is likely that oedema is the cause and recovery can be expected. However, in these cases a reducing course of steroids over 2–3 weeks may be given.

If the paralysis is immediate it indicates that the nerve has been severed or severely damaged by the injury. Surgical exploration of the facial nerve must be carried out as soon as the general condition of the patient permits.

The site of damage may be determined by a study of the function of the branches of the nerve with those still functioning lying proximal to the site of the injury:

1 Greater superficial petrosal nerve – lacrymation.

2 Chorda tympani – taste to the anterior two-thirds of the tongue.

3 Nerve to stapedius – stapedial reflex.

Ear surgery

In mastoid surgery, where bone is removed with a drill, the facial nerve is at risk, particularly if it is exposed or displaced by disease or if there is any anatomical abnormality. If the nerve is divided or damaged at surgery, immediate re-exploration must be performed and the damage repaired.

Parotid surgery

The facial nerve lies between the superficial and deep lobes of the parotid gland and is at risk during any procedure on the parotid. In the operation of superficial parotidectomy, the nerve is identified and all its branches are carefully dissected. It appears from a number of series that the nerve is at greater risk if a tumour is simply enucleated, as the site of the nerve and its branches has not been formally identified.

If the nerve has to be sacrificed for malignant

disease, primary grafting can be performed with good results.

External wounds

The nerve may, of course, be damaged in any external wound and repair can pose serious problems.

Mandibular branch of the facial nerve

This branch supplies the depressor of the lower lip, and section leaves an unsightly cosmetic defect. Its course is first into the neck and then it returns to the face at the anterior border of the masseter muscle and is, therefore, at risk in any incision below the mandible. An incision in this area must be made at least 2.5 cm below the mandible and this measurement should be made with the head in the normal position, not extended or turned to one side, or the normal anatomy will be distorted.

Inflammation

Herpes zoster oticus

Facial nerve paralysis accompanies the other features of the Ramsay Hunt syndrome – sensorineural deafness, vertigo, pain in the ear, and vesicles in the ear canal and mouth. The disease resolves slowly but the prognosis for the return of facial nerve function is only moderate. There is no specific treatment for the facial nerve paralysis and steroids should almost certainly not be given as they may allow the virus to spread to adjacent cranial nerves.

Bell's palsy

This is the commonest form of facial nerve paralysis.

Aetiology

This is not certain but it is thought that the nerve suffers viral inflammation and Bell's palsy may occur in small epidemics. The inflammation causes oedema of the nerve, but as it lies in a bony canal it cannot swell and pressure on the nerve occurs.

Symptoms

Facial paralysis, which may be rapid or slow in onset, and may be complete or incomplete. Pain in the ear may precede the onset of the paralysis.

Investigation

An examination to determine if the paralysis is complete, and nerve conduction studies will show the extent of nerve damage.

Treatment

Overall the prognosis is excellent for return of function – between 85 and 90 per cent. A bad prognostic feature is rapid onset of complete paralysis. If the paralysis is not complete, no treatment is needed but for some cases, and for cases of complete paralysis, a reducing course of steroids should be given.

In some centres, largely outside Great Britain, decompression of the facial nerve is performed on cases of complete paralysis of rapid onset.

Tumour: acoustic neuroma

This tumour of the sheath of the VIIIth nerve grows in

the internal auditory meatus where it causes compression of the facial nerve. Clinical facial paralysis occurs late, but evidence of facial nerve dysfunction can be obtained by a study of its branches.

1 Greater superficial petrosal nerve – decreased lacrymation.

2 Chorda tympani – decreased taste over the anterior two-thirds of the tongue tested by electrogustatometer.

3 Nerve to stapedius – abnormal stapedial reflex.

Intracranial

Any intracranial lesion – vascular, tumour, inflammatory or degenerative – can cause damage to the facial nerve nucleus or its upper motor neurone innervation. An upper motor neurone lesion can be distinguished from a lower, as there is bilateral upper motor neurone innervation of the forehead. In upper motor neurone lesions, therefore, the forehead is spared.

CHAPTER 6

HEAD AND NECK CANCER

Head and neck cancer poses a number of unique problems. First, the impact on the patient is very severe as the disease and surgery for it are visible; the head and neck cannot be hidden beneath clothing. The disease affects both the cosmetic appearance of the patient and his ability to talk and to eat. In reconstruction, the cosmetic and physiological results are equally important but, of course, to facilitate repair, ablation of disease must never be limited. The relatively recent introduction of free flaps, revascularised by microsurgical procedures, is likely to mean that much of the reconstructive work will be carried out by those who have a training in, and wide experience of, microvascular procedures.

The following comments on head and neck cancer management are generalisations. However, in management, generalisations are entirely inappropriate as a treatment programme must be planned for each individual patient.

A small number of patients will be treated by primary surgery, but a majority of head and neck patients will be treated first by a full course of radiotherapy. Surgery is reserved for recurrent or residual disease. This is because the results of 'salvage surgery' are no worse than those of primary surgery. Many patients will have been spared surgery which will inevitably affect, to some extent, the patient's appearance or his ability to talk or swallow.

If residual or recurrent disease is found at follow-up then three questions must be answered:

1 Is it possible to remove the tumour and to reconstruct the residual defect? Palliative surgery has little part to play in the management of incurable cases but, on occasions, may be justified.

2 Should the operation that is required be performed on this particular individual? The patient must be considered as a whole from all aspects: physical, psychological and social. It is essential to preserve and improve both the quantity and the quality of the patient's life.

3 Does the patient want the operation? Before reaching this decision the patient must be informed about all aspects of the surgery, both short- and long-term. A clear indication must be given as to how the operation will affect the patient's appearance and physiology, and how it will affect his quality of life. The patient must also be told that if surgery is declined then the disease will be fatal. It is only when a patient has all the information that informed consent to the surgical procedure can be given.

The operation is only a small part of the whole treatment of the patient, and preoperative preparation and post-operative care are equally important.

It is also extremely difficult to know how to inform a patient that the disease is serious enough to need radiotherapy and possibly surgery, without removing all hope of a cure. Unhappily, even today, many people believe that cancer is incurable, and cannot equate a diagnosis of cancer with the possibility of cure. In addition, many believe that a diagnosis of cancer means that the disease has spread throughout the body. Another grave problem is that to tell some patients that they have cancer is to destroy their quality of life, as it is spent in fear of a recurrence. A way out of this dilemma is to inform a patient that he has a pre-malignant or pre-cancerous condition which will develop into a cancer if not treated, but that radiotherapy should prevent this development and cause a regression of the tumour tissue. The patient can also be told at this stage that if all tumour tissue does not disappear surgery may be necessary, so that if surgery has to be performed the patient is at least partially prepared for it.

If after radiotherapy and surgery the patient has further untreatable and incurable disease, then either the patient or his relatives must be informed of the situation.

The aim must be in the future to inform everyone that certain forms of cancer can be cured, but it does not appear kind to place this education programme on the shoulders of an individual patient.

Patients with head and neck cancer do not die from distant metastases, and their death is from local disease and is often slow, painful and extremely distressing to the patient, his relatives and his medical attendants. Enormous sympathy and support is required, and terminal care must be of the very highest standard in the relief of physical and psychological suffering.

Individual Tumours

A majority of head and neck tumours have been discussed in the individual chapters, but details of the management of a solitary lump in the neck must be given as to incise a metastatic carcinomatous node in the neck is to condemn a patient to death.

Midline swellings

These are rare and the only one commonly met is the thyroglossal cyst. This cyst may present during the course of an upper respiratory tract infection and may then be the site of repeated inflammatory swellings. The diagnosis is made by asking the patient first to open his mouth, and then to protrude the tongue, which will cause the cyst to move upwards as it is tethered to the tongue at the foramen caecum.

When excised surgically the centre of the body of the hyoid bone must be removed as the tract loops up behind the body or occasionally passes through it. If this is not done then a part of the tract will be left *in situ* and recurrence will be almost inevitable.

A diagnostic pitfall is that the 'thyroglossal cyst' may in fact be the only portion of the functioning thyroid tissue possessed by the patient. An examination of the neck will reveal if a thyroid gland is present, but if there is any doubt then a thyroid scan must be performed.

Diagnosis of a Lateral Neck Mass

It has been said that there is no condition more easy to

examine yet more difficult to diagnose.

Specific swellings

Salivary tumour

Tumours of the parotid are much more common than
those of the submandibular salivary gland (9 : 1), but
whereas parotid tumours are almost invariably benign
(9 : 1) tumours of the submandibular gland are most
frequently malignant in a similar ratio.

In addition, there are islands of ectopic salivary
tissue around the mouth and throat, and a common site
for the development of a tumour is lateral to the tonsil.
If a patient presents with a 'painless quinsy' one must
suspect that this is an ectopic salivary tumour.

Submandibular gland

Stones commonly develop in the duct of the submandibular salivary gland and give rise to the classic
symptoms of pain and swelling of the gland when the
patient salivates. X-ray studies including intra-oral
views will show the presence of a stone and, if it is far
forward in the duct, then it may be removed under
either local or general anaesthetic. However, if the
stone is far back, or if there are many stones, then the
submandibular salivary gland may need to be removed, and in the incision the mandibular branch of
the facial nerve must be avoided. However, if the
symptoms of pain and swelling are absent, then a
submandibular salivary gland mass must be assumed
to be a tumour. It must also be presumed that it is
malignant.

Treatment is by wide excision biopsy followed by

radiotherapy as appropriate, but the cure rates for these tumours are relatively poor.

Parotid

Although the majority of parotid gland tumours are benign, those which are malignant infrequently show the stigmata of malignancy which are rapid growth, pain and involvement of the facial nerve. The management of a parotid mass is the subject of much heated debate.

An open biopsy should not be performed, as to close the wound after biopsy leads to the seeding of tumour within the tissues of the neck and frozen section is notoriously inaccurate. Fine-needle aspiration is difficult to interpret and, although it is easier to interpret a specimen taken by wide-bore needle, this may still not be representative and there is a slight but significant risk of tumour seeding.

There are two alternatives: first to enucleate the tumour, and second to perform a superficial parotidectomy. There are several arguments against enucleation followed by radiotherapy, namely that the surface of a pleomorphic adenoma, which is the commonest benign parotid tumour, is bosselated, and in an enucleation it is certain that some of the bosses will be broken off and tumour fragments will be left in the wound leading to a recurrence rate of 40–50 per cent without radiotherapy. Pleomorphic adenomas have some malignant potential and it has been suggested that to irradiate these tumours may provoke rather than prevent malignant change. In addition, the facial nerve appears to be more at risk in an enucleation than in a superficial parotidectomy where the nerve is exposed and dissected.

Despite some support for enucleation and radiotherapy, a majority of surgeons suggest that a superficial parotidectomy should be performed with exposure and preservation of the facial nerve. The aim of this procedure is to remove the parotid tumour with an intact, complete cuff of normal parotid tissue, and if this aim is achieved then the operation should be successful. However, the situation of the tumour in the parotid gland often means that during the dissection the capsule of the gland is exposed commonly where it lies on the facial nerve, and if the capsule is seen then, in effect, an enucleation only has been performed. Where the capsule has been exposed then the patient must be considered for postoperative radiotherapy to reduce the recurrence rate to acceptable levels.

Branchial cyst

This congenital cyst often presents in childhood or early adult life during the course of an upper respiratory tract infection but, on occasions, may present late in life and will then provide a difficult, diagnostic problem. The swelling lies at the junction of the lower two-thirds and upper one-third of the sternomastoid muscle, and one-third of it projects in front of the muscle with two-thirds deep to it.

Carotid body tumour

This is often known as the potato tumour as it is extremely slow growing and arises in chemodectoma tissue of the carotid body at the bifurcation of the carotid arteries. These hard tumours can be moved in an anteroposterior direction but not up and down, and it is vitally important not to biopsy one of these in error as the bleeding may be severe. An arteriogram should be performed which shows the classic 'wine-glass' abnormality, with the carotids separated with vascular tissue in between. It is probably wise to perform an arteriogram on any tumour so closely related to the carotid arteries. Surgery is extremely difficult and may well require carotid arterial by-pass and/or grafting.

Pharyngeal pouch

The aetiology and management of a pharyngeal pouch has been discussed in the section on dysphagia and these, on occasions, may present as an intermittent swelling, usually on the left side of the neck.

Laryngocoele

This should be easy to diagnose as it occurs commonly in those who play brass instruments. During the playing of the instrument the vocal cords are closed and in effect a 'valsalva manoeuvre' is performed with a great rise in the upper laryngeal and pharyngeal pressure. This dilates a laryngeal ventricle which lies between the false and true cords, and this appears in the neck as an air-filled swelling. X-rays will confirm the diagnosis and the treatment is by surgery.

Neuroma

Neuromas of the major cranial nerves in the neck are rare and may often only be diagnosed at surgery.

Lymph node

As mentioned earlier one of the most serious crimes that a surgeon can commit is to cut into a lymph node involved by metastatic carcinoma, as this will reduce the already small cure rate of these patients to nil. A lymph node may be involved by acute inflammation, which is usually easy to diagnose as the node is hot and painful and there is almost invariably an obvious focus of infection. The glands from chronic inflammation such as tuberculosis are often not diffuse and matted. If a patient with a lymphoma presents with a solitary node in the neck, without involvement of other nodes or other node groups, then he is unlikely to have the systemic symptoms associated with this group of diseases. An additional problem unique to head and neck cancer is that a minute symptomless primary tumour may present with a large metastatic node. It has been said that the patient who presents with symptoms from his primary is much more fortunate than the patient with a symptom-free primary tumour. This is because the symptoms will lead to the primary being identified and will effectively rule out the danger of having the lymph node inappropriately biopsied.

Management of a Solitary Neck Mass

It is usually easy to identify and to treat the specific masses mentioned above, and also to exclude an acute inflammatory node.

When these pathologies have been excluded the patient must then have a lymph node involved by chronic inflammation, lymphoma or metastatic carcinoma. Assuming an absence of symptoms to draw the attention of the doctor to a primary tumour, all patients must have a full ENT/head and neck examination to attempt to find the 'occult primary tumour'. If a tumour cannot be found in the clinic then it is often necessary to carry out a full examination under anaesthetic with blind biopsies of the nasopharynx where submucosal, invisible and impalpable tumours may occur. Bronchoscopy and oesophagoscopy will also be performed.

If a tumour has not been found, and if the node is low in the neck, a search should be performed for a possible primary below the clavicles, including a chest X-ray for a bronchial tumour and a barium meal for a gastric lesion.

If investigations are still negative, then the neck must be explored. The majority of 'head and neck' surgeons prepare the patient for a radical neck dissection. They then expose the mass through an incision which can be extended into one through which a radical neck dissection can be performed. Isolating the mass from other tissues, a biopsy and frozen section can then be carried out. If histology shows chronic inflammation or a lymphoma, the node alone will be removed. However, if a metastatic squamous carcinoma is found then a radical neck dissection should be performed, removing all the soft tissue between the platysma and prevertebral fascia including the sterno-mastoid muscle and internal jugular vein but leaving behind the carotid arteries and vagus and phrenic nerves.

There is some dispute as to whether this is the ideal treatment regime, and some suggest that removal of the gland followed by radiotherapy provides an equally good treatment. However, in patients with an 'occult primary' the primary tumour will manifest itself in 50 per cent, whereas in 50 per cent it will never be found. In patients who do develop an obvious primary then radiotherapy is the first line of potentially curative treatment, and if the whole neck has been irradiated to a relatively low dose, then further radiotherapy for cure of the primary cannot easily be given (see Figure 6.1).

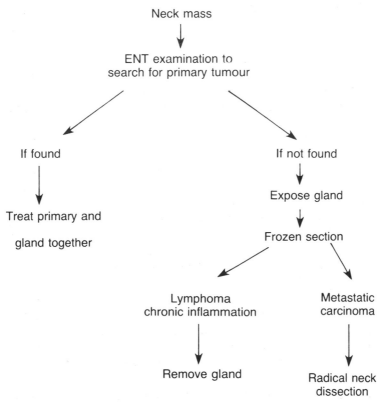

Figure 6.1

If a patient with a head and neck malignancy has developed a metastatic node then taken overall the cure rate is between 25 and 40 per cent. If an incisional biopsy of the node has been carried out then this cure rate will fall to 0 per cent.

A further development which may significantly change and improve this problem, is the development of fine-needle aspiration biopsy of suspicious neck nodes which can be carried out without significant risk of seeding of tumour in the tissues of the neck and will readily distinguish between a metastatic squamous carcinoma and other pathologies. At present this technique is not widely available but, if and when it is, the problem of the management of a solitary neck node will be much simplified and improved.

INDEX

Achalasia of the Cardia   78
Acoustic Neuroma   158,167
Acute Epiglottitis   89
Acute Otitis Media   14
Adenoidectomy
   Complications   22
   Indications   13
   The Operation   23
Adenoids   1,13,35
   Ear Disease   14
   Nasal Obstruction   13
Antro Choanal Polyp   53
Audiometry   117
Aural Polyp   140

Bell's Palsy   167
Benign Positional Vertigo   160
Branchial Cyst   175
Bulbar Palsy   77

Caldwell-Luc Operation   53
Caloric Tests   123
Carbon Dioxide Laser   28,93
Carcinoma of Maxilla   37
Carcinoma of the
Oesophagus   74
Carcinoma of the Post Nasal
Space   39
Carotid Body Tumour   175
Choanal Atresia   28

Cholesteatoma   135
Chorda Tympani   165,168
Chronic Suppurative Otitis
Media   130,154
   Safe   130
   Unsafe   134
Cochlea   116
Colon Transplant   76
Congenital Laryngeal
Stridor   99
Croup   88

Deaf Children's Clinic   149
Deafness   116
Deafness in Children   146
Deviated Nasal Septum   26
Diffuse Oesophageal
Spasm   79
Diplacusis   157
Diptheria   91
Dysphagia   67

Ear Drum   110
   Rupture   130
   Scarring   139
   Viral Myringitis   128
Ear – Examination   109
Ear Syringing   128
Electrocochleography   149
Electronystagmography   122

Endolymphatic Sac   158
Endotracheal Intubation –
Prolonged   86
Ethmoid Sinuses   46
Ethmoid Sinusitis Acute   46
External Auditory
Meatus   109
   Atresia   125
   Infection   125
   Furuncle   126
   Wax   128
External Otitis   125

Facial Fractures   62
Facial Nerve Paralysis   164
Fine Needle Aspiration
Biopsy   180
Fluid in the Middle Ear
   Signs   20
   Treatment   21
Foreign Body in Oesophagus
   Complications – Ingested
Corrosives   72
   Complications –
Mediastinitis   71
Frontal Sinus   43
Frontal Sinusitis Acute   43
Frontal Sinusitis After
Intracranial Complications   44
Frontal Sinusitis
Recurrent   44
Frontal Sinus Mucocele   45
Fronto Ethmoidectomy   44

Glandular Fever   66
Globus Hystericus   80
Glue Ear   18
Greater Superficial Petrosal
Nerve   165,168
Grommet   22

Haematoma of Nasal
Septum   61

Haemorrhage
   Classification   8
   Management of Post
Tonsillectomy   11
   Primary   8
   Reactionary   8
   Secondary   9
   Signs   9
Haemotympanum   140
Head and Neck Cancer   169
Hearing Aids   151
Hearing – Tests   110
Herpes Zoster Oticus   155,166
Hoarseness   81

Impedance Audiometry   117
Inner Ear Function –
Tests   117
Inner Ear Infection
   Bacterial   154
   Viral   155
Inner Ear Trauma   149,152,
Inner Ear – Vascular
Accident   153
Labyrinthectomy   146,158
Laryngitis
   Acute   88
   Chronic   91
Laryngocoele   176
Laryngomalacia   99
Laryngoscopy   81
Larynx   81
   Allergy   98
   Burns   87
   Carcinoma   94
   Cysts   82
   External Trauma   85
   Foreign Body   87
   Juvenile Papillomatosis   92
   Leukoplakia   93
   Rheumatoid Arthritis   99
   Subglottic Stenosis   83
   Trauma   84

Lymph Node in Neck   177
  Management   177

Macbeth Operation   45
Malignant Granuloma   36
Mastoidectomy   138
Maxillary Sinus   48
Maxillary Sinusitis
  Acute   49
  Chronic   51
  Recurrent Acute   50
Maxillary Sinus Washout   52
Ménière's Disease   156
Meningitis   148,154
Middle Ear
  Adhesions   140
  Anatomy   113
  Blood   140
  Fluid   139
  Physiology   114
  Polypi   140
Myringoplasty   134

Nasal Allergy
  Paroxysmal   30
  Perennial   31
Nasal Fibro-angioma   35
Nasal Injuries   61
Nasal Mucosa
  Allergy   30
  Inflammation   29
Nasal Obstruction   26
Nasal Packing   57
Nasal Polypi   34,47
Nasal Tumours   35
Neck Dissection – Radical   178
Nerve to Stapedius   165,168
Noise Induced Hearing
Loss   150
Nose Bleed   54
  Recurrent   60
  Examination   25
  Foreign Body   28

Nystagmus   120

Oesophageal
  Atresia   68
  Foreign Body   69
  Avascular Necrosis   141
  Dislocation   141
Otosclerosis   142
Ototoxic Drugs   156

Palatal Myoclonus   162
Paracusis   142
Parotidectomy –
Superficial   174
Parotid Surgery   165
Parotid Tumours   174
Paterson, Brown-Kelly
Syndrome   74
Pharyngeal Pouch   77,176
Pharyngitis
  Bacterial   64
  Viral   63
Pharyngolaryngectomy   76
Pinna   109
  Absence   123
  Diseases   123
  Infection   124
  Trauma   124
Positional Tests   122
Post Nasal Packing   58
Presbyacusis   150
Pseudo Bulbar Palsy   77

Quinsy   3,65

Ramsay Hunt
Syndrome   155,166
Recurrent Laryngeal Nerve
Paralysis   83,97
Recurrent Respiratory
Papillomatosis   92
Reflux Oesophagitis   73
Respiratory Failure   102

Rinne Test   111
Round Window Membrane
Rupture   152
Rubella   147

Sensorineural Deafness   144
Serous Otitis Media   17,21
Sinuses and Sinusitis   40
Sinusitis
  Pain   41
  Sinus Rupture   41
Sore Throat   63
Sphenoid Sinus   42
Stomach Pull-up   76
Stridor   81
Stuart Tube   76
Submandibular Gland
  Stone in Duct   173
  Tumours   174
Submucous Resection of the
Nasal Septum (SMR)   26
Syringing of Ear   128

Temporal Bone Fracture   164
Throat Examination   63
Thrush   67
Thyroglossal Cyst   172
Tinnitus   161,162
Tinnitus Maskers   163
Tinnitus
  Objective   162
  Subjective   162
Tonsillectomy   2
  Contraindications   6
  For Histology   5
  Indications   3
  The Operation   8

Tonsillitis   2,3,65
Tonsils   1
  Size   5
Tracheostomy   99
  Care   105
  Complications   106
  Indications   100
  The Operation   103
  Tube   105
  Tube Fixation   105
Transitional Cell Papilloma of
Nose   35
Traumatic Rupture of Ear
Drum   130
Trotter's Method to Control
Nose Bleed   55
Tympanometry   117
Tympanoplasty   134

Upper Airway
Obstruction   100

Vagus – Lesions   96
Vaso-motor Rhinitis   33
Vertebro Basilar
Insufficiency   160
Vestibular Apparatus   116
Vestibular Function   120
Vestibular Function Clinical
Tests   120
Vestibular Neuronitis   159
Vocal Cord – Webs   82
Vertigo   145

Waldeyer's Ring   1
Wax in Ear   128
Weber Test   112